Legal Aspects of
General Dental Practice

For Elsevier:

Commissioning Editor: Michael Parkinson

Development Editor: Janice Urquhart

Project Manager: Gail Wright

Design Direction: Stewart Larking

Illustrator: David Gardner

Legal Aspects of General Dental Practice

Len D'Cruz
BDS LLM LDSRCS(Eng) DipFOd MFGDP
General Dental Practitioner, Dento-legal Advisor, Dental Protection, London, UK

With contributions from
Simon Mills
MB BCh BAO (Dubl.) BCL (NUI) MSc (Lond.)
Barrister at Law, Medical Practitioner, Law Library, Four Courts, Dublin, Ireland

David Holmes
Shepherd and Wedderburn, Solicitors, Edinburgh, UK

Foreword by
Kevin Lewis
BDS LDS RCS
Dental Director, Dental Protection, London, UK

Series Editor
F. J. Trevor Burke
Professor of Dental Primary Care, University of Birmingham School of Dentistry, Birmingham, UK

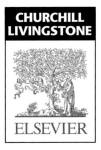

Edinburgh London New York Oxford Philadelphia St Louis Sydney Toronto 2006

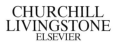

CHURCHILL
LIVINGSTONE
ELSEVIER

First published 2006

ISBN 0 443 10038 1

British Library Cataloguing in Publication Data
A catalogue record for this book is available from the British Library

Library of Congress Cataloging in Publication Data
A catalog record for this book is available from the Library of Congress

Notice
Neither the Publisher nor the Authors assume any responsibility for any loss or injury and/or damage to persons or property arising out of or related to any use of the material contained in this book. It is the responsibility of the treating practitioner, relying on independent expertise and knowledge of the patient, to determine the best treatment and method of application for the patient.

The Publisher

ELSEVIER your source for books, journals and multimedia in the health sciences
www.elsevierhealth.com

The publisher's policy is to use paper manufactured from sustainable forests

Working together to grow libraries in developing countries
www.elsevier.com | www.bookaid.org | www.sabre.org

ELSEVIER **BOOK AID** International Sabre Foundation

Printed in China

Contents

Foreword

Life in a busy dental practice can be complicated enough without the additional impact of ever-increasing legislation and bureaucracy that practitioners and their staff must deal with.

Dentistry is of course not alone in facing this problem, as any restaurateur, teacher, policeman, factory owner or business person will tell you; but every business or profession must understand how essentially the same laws assume their meaning and application in their own individual circumstances. The English laws of tort and contract, or the legislation relating to data protection, were not of course written with dentists in mind.

It is not possible, in a work such as this, to throw light on every dark corner of dental practice, nor to examine the application of every piece of UK legislation to it. Len D'Cruz has therefore chosen to focus upon the main pillars of the legal aspects of dental practice in the UK, and mostly upon English law. He covers the legal basis for professional standards (including negligence and serious professional misconduct), and the ethical and legal aspects of consent and confidentiality. Against that background, he has provided detailed sections on record keeping (both manual and electronic), complaints systems and report writing. For good measure, he provides a brief overview of the UK legal system which provides a helpful introduction for the reader who is new to this subject.

His decision not to become deflected into the massive areas of Employment Law and Health & Safety Legislation is vindicated by the time and space it has allowed to explore the chosen areas, and Len D'Cruz's passion for his subject is self-evident.

The law can seem very academic and distant from the interface between a patient and members of the dental team, but in fact it permeates most, if not all, of the everyday working procedures in the dental practice environment.

This is made clear by the regular practical illustrations of how the law would apply to familiar situations and dilemmas in modern dental practice, that are provided throughout the text. By the constructive use of such illustrations, Len D'Cruz has provided both pace and momentum as the reader discovers that the law really can be both interesting and relevant to those in dental practice.

Kevin Lewis

Preface

This book aims to provide the basic principles of law relating to general dental practice for final-year students, vocational dental practitioners as well as busy general dental practitioners. Working for Dental Protection, it became increasingly clear that whilst many dentists have a general understanding of such fundamental issues as consent, confidentiality and clinical negligence, there was no one place they could find more detail and practical guidance in the application of those principles. The defence organisations all produce risk management publications and in the case of Dental Protection this is quite extensive but I felt there was a need to locate these in one source.

The law is stimulating, challenging and sometimes provocatively odd, but keeping abreast of it all can be daunting. I have tried as far as possible to state these principles as simply as possible, mindful that new cases and statutes may change the interpretation of things even as fundamental as consent.

Some readers may have wished for other topics to have been covered but I have confined myself to those areas most often enquired about from my own work as a dento-legal advisor and speaker at various postgraduate meetings around the UK.

I would like to sincerely thank my wife Anne and sons for their patience, understanding and unconditional (well almost) support and especially to Simon, who was born whilst this book was being written, and who kept me company on many an early-morning writing session.

My apologies to Margaret Grew, who was looking for 'some romance' within the pages of this book. There is none but maybe next time…

I have endeavoured to state the law as at February 2005.

L. T. D'C.
2005
London

Abbreviations

BSA	Business Services Authority
CFSMS	Counter Fraud and Security Management Service
CHAI	Commission of Healthcare Audit and Improvement
CHI	Commission for Health Improvement
CHRE	Council for Healthcare Regulatory Excellence
CPD	continuing professional development
CPR	Civil Procedure Rules
CRHP	Council for the Regulation of Health Care Professionals
EPR	electronic patient record
GA	general anaesthesia
GDC	General Dental Council
GMC	General Medical Council
HSC	Health Service Commissioner
IR[ME]R 2000	Ionising Radiation (Medical Exposure) Regulations 2000
NCAA	National Clinical Assessment Authority
NICE	National Institute for Clinical Excellence
NPSA	National Patient Safety Agency
PACE	Police and Criminal Evidence Act 1984
PAERS	Patient Access Electronic Record System
PCC	Professional Conduct Committee
PCDs	professionals complementary to dentistry
PCT	primary care trust
SIDS	sudden infant death syndrome
TBBD	temporary brittle bone disease
TQM	total quality management
VDPs	vocational dental practitioners

Legal structures and processes that impact in general dental practice

1

The starting point of any book on dento-legal perspectives in general practice ought to be an overview of the legal system, as well as how healthcare fits into the regulatory framework.

Even before this it is important to provide an understanding of what dental law is and why it is important. In their opus *Medical Law*, Kennedy and Grubb[1] describe medical law as being a subset of human rights. Law in its widest sense is a form of social control which is set down by the state in the form of rules and is enforced through the courts and the legal system.

Running through dental law are two key themes—the rights of patients and others, and the duties of the dentist. Much of a dentist's relationship with patients is embodied by these two themes, which sometimes conflict and are underpinned both by statute and common law, as well as a set of guiding principles of ethical and professional behaviour.

FOUR PRINCIPLES OF HEALTHCARE ETHICS

Four principles of healthcare ethics have been identified[2] and summarised by Hope et al (see further reading at end of chapter), and are useful tools for dentists facing ethical or moral dilemmas in practice.

1. Respect for patient autonomy

Autonomy is the capacity to think and decide, and then act on the basis of such thought and decision, freely and independently. Respect for a patient's autonomy means giving the information necessary to allow that patient to make informed decisions, and then to respect those decisions and follow them even when the professional may believe they are the wrong decisions. The flip side of this self-determination is paternalism, where a dentist makes a decision without necessarily taking the patient's wishes into consideration.

2. Beneficence: promotion of what is best for the patient

This is a fundamental aspect of dental care for patients and the duty of the dentist is to steer the patient into what is best for them. What is best is an objective assessment of that patient's needs and this would in most cases chime with what the patient wants under the principle of autonomy. The two principles conflict when a competent patient makes a decision which is patently not in their best interests.

3. Non-maleficence: avoiding harm

It is a well-recognised maxim in healthcare that firstly we should do no harm. Thus, treatment provided should have more benefits than harmful effects, and this is a significant consideration when elective cosmetic dentistry is involved.

4. Justice

This is a broader, policy-based principle which attempts to distribute the finite resources of time and money in a fair and equitable manner. This means that patients in similar situations should have access to the same care, whilst also recognising that care for one type of patient will influence the resources available for others.

These principles of practice have been incorporated in the General Dental Council's guidance 'Standards for dental professionals':

1. Putting patients first and acting to protect them.
2. Respecting patients' dignity and choices.
3. Protecting the confidentiality of patients' information.
4. Cooperating with other members of the dental team and other healthcare colleagues in the interests of patients.
5. Maintaining your professional knowledge and competence.
6. Being trustworthy.

Thus dental law will encompass ethical and professional responsibilities as well as adherence to the law of the land. The sanctions for breaking these two different codes are sometimes quite different. For example, being found legally liable for civil negligence will result in the dentist, or more often their indemnity organisation, paying damages to the patient. Being found guilty of professional misconduct by the General Dental Council could result in the dentist's erasure from the Register and perhaps an end to their career in dentistry.

BRANCHES OF LAW

The law (Fig. 1.1) can be divided up into public and private law (more commonly known as civil law). Public law involves the government or instruments of government, whilst private law is concerned with disputes between individuals or companies.

Administrative law controls how, for example, local health authorities should operate and how decisions they make may be challenged by a judicial review. Public law encompasses criminal law, where the state takes the role of prosecuting a law-breaker and enforcing punishments.

Private law has many branches, and the law of tort, contract law and employment law are of immediate relevance to dental practice.

A tort is a civil wrong which is actionable and occurs even when there is no contract between two people. It exists because in a civil society one person can owe someone else a duty of care, even if they are complete strangers. When that duty of care has been breached, damages can be obtained by the injured party.

Contract law is about the rules concerning the identification, regulation and enforcement of agreements. These agreements cover many aspects of everyday life, such as shopping, travelling on a train or buying a meal in a restaurant. In dentistry, contracts are drawn up between practice owners and associates. They also exist between dentists and laboratories, and between practices and suppliers. Many contracts are not written down, but when they are, contracts serve as important documents that protect each party and define the terms of a relationship.

Employment law for practice owners is an ever-developing field, and many changes have occurred in employment legislation that impact directly and very significantly on general practice. Any dentist who needs advice on a specific issue relating to the employment, conduct or dismissal of a member of staff should contact their professional organisation, their indemnity provider or a lawyer.

SOURCES OF LAW

The two main sources of law are statute law (which would include European legislation) and common or judge-made law.

Statute law

This encompasses Acts of Parliament introduced by the government in power, in response either to party policy, the media or pressure groups. The government may consult interested parties and

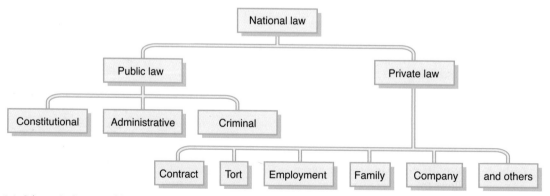

Fig. 1.1 Schematic diagram of the branches of law.

the public through 'green' and 'white' papers before drafting the legislation into a Bill. When parliamentary time allows, the Bill is introduced into the House of Commons and follows various stages—a first reading, a second reading, a committee stage, a third stage which follows the report stage and then (if there are no objections) a vote on whether the Bill should be accepted. The Bill is then sent to the House of Lords, which has no power to veto but only amend, although they can delay a Bill for up to a year. The Bill is then sent to the Queen for her assent, whereupon it becomes an Act and passes on to the statute books.

Common law

Common law is so-called in England because historically judges were sent by the King around the country from London to hear cases and pass judgement in disputes. The judges decided cases on local customs which varied around the country, but gradually, as the judges discussed their cases together back in Westminster, they formulated the best custom and practice to follow and these became 'common' to all parts of the country.

An essential part of today's common law is the doctrine of precedent. This is where a decision of a court may be binding on future courts in a similar case. The circumstances which make it binding depend on the position of the court in the court hierarchy and whether the material facts are the same.

In terms of court hierarchy in England, the highest court in the land is the House of Lords, and all the decisions it makes bind all lower courts below—the Court of Appeal, the divisional courts, the Crown Court (in criminal cases) and the High Court (in civil cases), and magistrates and county courts.

The doctrine of precedent is important in clinical negligence claims, whilst in ethical and moral dilemmas it is useful to have a House of Lords decision. Such matters may include the right to live, as in the case of conjoined twins or consent issues of refusing life-saving treatment.

The doctrine of precedent allows a degree of certainty in the law, such that by following a previous decision a lawyer can advise a client properly in terms of the likely outcome of a case. Precedent also allows the law to reflect changes in society and thinking, which makes it quite a flexible way of changing the law. There are concomitant disadvantages, such as judges making apparently conflicting decisions even when the facts of a case are similar, or when precedent legally binds lower courts even when a decision was bad or harsh.

EQUITY

Historically, the law of equity (or fairness) arose out of dissatisfaction with the remedies available from the common law, which could only offer damages, normally money, to compensate a wronged party. In some cases it may be more appropriate to use different remedies. Today the main equitable remedies of injunctions, specific performance, rescission and rectification remain important. Injunctions can be ordered against a violent patient from attending the practice, forbidding them from entering or coming near the premises. They also can be used in employment law to maintain confidential information or trade secrets when employees leave the business.

THE GENERAL DENTAL COUNCIL

Parliament has allowed dentistry, through various Acts (the latest being the Dentists Act 1984), to regulate itself, primarily by maintaining a register of dental professionals who are competent and fit to practise. Self regulation is a cherished aspect of dentistry as a profession. However, this has come under severe pressure in recent years with scandals, such as the Shipman, Ledward and the Bristol heart babies cases, dominating the headlines and undermining public confidence and trust in the ability of healthcare professions to govern themselves. The remit of the General Dental Council (GDC) is primarily to protect patients and the professional status and reputation of the dental profession, and this is clear from the Act itself:

The Council shall, in exercise of its functions under this Act, have a general concern—

a) *to promote, at all stages, high standards of education in all aspects of dentistry*
b) *to promote high standards of professional conduct, performance and practice amongst persons registered under the Act.*

The Dentists Act 1984, Part I, section 1 (2) as amended by Amendment Order 2005

It does this by maintaining a dental register and issuing guidance on standards of dental practice and conduct. It also quality assures dental undergraduate education through its Education Committee.

The actions normally taken by regulatory bodies are to protect members of the public from the professional activities of a dentist, hygienist or therapist who may either cause harm, or undertake treatment which falls short of the expected standards which would have been provided by their peers. If patients are looking for the quick resolution of complaints, an explanation or an apology, the GDC route is not the one to take. However, some patients feel the need to 'punish' the wrongdoer, and the removal of the dentist's name from the register would be seen in that light. It is important to remember that the GDC does not aim to punish dentists, and when a dentist's name is removed from the register following an inquiry, this action is taken solely to protect the public.

Protected title

The Dentists Act gives statutory protection to the title 'dentist', as well as the actual practice of dentistry. Unlike in medicine where there is no legislative restriction on who can treat patients or provide medical or health-related service, it is a criminal offence to carry out the practice of dentistry if not qualified or registered to do so, although a registered doctor can practise dentistry.

> *No person shall take or use any title or description implying that he is a registered dentist unless he is a registered dentist*

The Dentists Act 1984, Part IV **39** (2)

Registration

Entry to the dental register is based on primary qualifications set out in the Dentists Act 1984, the commonest route being via a dental degree from a UK dental school. The United Kingdom's membership of the European Union has brought the freedom of movement of workers across borders. Under EU legislation, EU nationals who have carried out their dental training in the new EU countries will be entitled to apply for full registration with the GDC.

Professions complementary to dentistry (PCDs) also have various routes on to the register, with hygienists and therapists currently on the register and other classes (such as dental technicians, dental nurses and orthodontic auxiliaries) to be included in 2006 when the Section 60 order is passed.

Reform

The GDC has jurisdiction over dentists in England, Scotland, Wales and Northern Ireland, and whilst the legal systems and NHS structures have continued to develop independently in the devolved administrations, Parliament still reserves power over the regulation of the professions.

The Kennedy Report, following the Bristol babies scandal,[3] called for a system which 'needs the widest involvement of professionals, of the principal employer and of the public...An effective system of professional regulation must be owned collectively. Further, it needs an independence from the professions and from government which allows it to act in the public's interest'.

Reform is coming in the shape of a new organisation that will oversee the decisions made by the GDC — the Council for Healthcare Regulatory Excellence. It is also coming in the shape of reforms of the GDC itself. As the first step towards increased public involvement and a faster, more transparent operating system in the council, the Dentists Act 1984 Amended Order 2002 (SI 2002 No.3926) was made under section 60 of the Health Act 1992. This amended the GDC into a smaller Council with a higher proportion of lay members, made continuing professional development (CPD) compulsory and enabled the Council to set up a new independent 'Fitness to Practise' Panel to hear conduct and health cases.

Further changes to the regulation of the profession will occur through a second section 60 order in 2005. This was drafted in July 2004 and was intended to be put before the Privy Council by the government and signed by the Queen in January 2005. This was then delayed until July 2005 at the earliest, with the likelihood that its provisions will not enable the GDC to make any changes until 2006 and possibly 2007 for aspects relating to registration of PCDs (professionals complementary to dentistry).

This section 60 order is intended to modernise the GDC's fitness-to-practise procedures for dealing with misconduct and ill health amongst dental professionals, and to introduce new procedures to tackle problems of poor performance.

The structure and sanctions of the GDC have hitherto been a blunt instrument to tackle issues of poor performance. A dentist's conduct may give rise to concerns, but if that conduct does not cross the threshold of serious professional misconduct, the GDC has no powers to address such shortcomings, which may be, for example, in terms of attitude, aptitude or communication skills.

Other changes that will occur in 2005 and beyond with the section 60 order are:

1. Removal of restrictions on dental body corporates.
2. Dental hygienists and therapists enabled to develop new skills within their training and competence.
3. Regulation of other PCDs, such as dental nurses, dental technicians, clinical dental technicians and orthodontic therapists.
4. Mandatory indemnity cover for all registrants.

Private patients' complaints scheme

The reforms in the pipeline are quite wide-ranging and will also establish a private patients' complaints scheme, funded by the GDC but separate from it. This has always been a cause for concern both for the dentist and the public. Private patient complaints often do not amount to the suggestion that the registrant's conduct would amount to serious professional misconduct, and therefore the GDC would have no reason to consider it. The only other route for the patient was a civil claim in negligence.

For the dentists themselves, the GDC's involvement was an unwelcome and unnecessary addition to the stress of receiving a complaint.

The impetus for a private patients' complaints scheme came also from the Office of Fair Trading (OFT), which had looked at dentistry following a super-complaint from the Consumers Association in 2001.

The scheme will mirror the NHS complaints scheme, with emphasis on supporting practices to resolve complaints locally. Where this is not possible, the new body will investigate and resolve complaints. As part of this local structure, there will also be GDC-recognised Practitioner Advice

and Support Schemes (PASS) which may also look at a broad range of concerns about a dental professional, with panel membership drawn locally from the Health Authority and local practitioners.

Disciplinary function (see Appendix 1)

In common with the General Medical Council, the GDC has been reviewing its procedures, primarily in response to concerns from the public that misconduct among dental professionals was going unpunished, with dentists 'looking after their own'. The review is also in response to the introduction of the Human Rights Act 1998. The lack of transparency and the seeming injustice of the Council being the 'prosecutor' and 'adjudicator' in disciplinary matters has resulted in the establishment of a separate fitness-to-practise panel whose members are appointed and not members of the GDC.

Initial stage of complaint receipt

The first stage in the procedure is the receipt of a complaint in writing. This complaint or information may come from a wide range of sources, such as a patient, another registrant, an employer or health authority, or the police.

The Council is informed automatically by the police if a dentist has been convicted in the UK of a criminal offence. The Council can consider any criminal conviction, including offences not directly connected to the practice of dentistry or which occurred while the dentist was not registered.

This has two significant implications. Offences such as fraud, assault, drink-driving and theft, even if unconnected with dentistry, will be reported to the GDC if they result in a criminal conviction. This also means that dental students, convicted of an offence whilst undergraduates, have found themselves facing GDC disciplinary proceedings as soon as they apply to become registered following graduation.

As part of the registration procedure, a dentist will need to satisfy the Registrar that they are fit to be registered, both in terms of health and character. A number of dental students have fallen foul of this regulation. A criminal conviction, or even a caution, will come to the attention of the Dean of the dental school, and university authorities are obliged to reveal the details of such episodes in their statement of good character to the GDC. In any case, under regulations in force since 2002, a dentist wishing to work in the NHS (even as a vocational dental practitioner [VDP]) must declare any convictions or police cautions to the Health Authority, who may then decline to issue an NHS contract number depending on the circumstances.

Patients' complaints no longer need to be supported by a statutory declaration or an affidavit—a legal process that in the past hindered patients' access to the Council's disciplinary procedures.

NHS or private complaint

On receipt of the complaint, the GDC's professional standards officers will decide whether the complaint is one that they can deal with. The first consideration is whether treatment was provided under the NHS or private contract. If the treatment was provided under the NHS, the GDC will usually consider referring the patient back to the Health Authority/Primary Care Trust (England and Wales), Health Board (Scotland) or Health and Social Services Board (Northern Ireland). The aim would be to try and resolve the complaint at a local level. Whilst a private patients' complaints scheme remains to be established, many more patients who have received private dental care will address their complaints directly to the GDC without using the practice-based complaints procedure.

Serious professional misconduct

In 1987, the Judicial Committee of the Privy Council decided that in establishing 'serious professional misconduct', the 'Council should establish conduct connected with his profession in which the dentist concerned has fallen short, by omission or commission, of the standards of conduct expected among dentists and that falling short, as is established, should be serious'.

Cases coming before the conduct committee vary widely in nature and circumstances. Some cases recently considered include Example 1–5.[i]

The emphasis on the seriousness of the misconduct is one of the key changes to take place. The aim in the new system will be to look at what past behaviour (i.e. the incident or complaint that

Example 1

A dentist, in a single case brought to the GDC, had placed implants and fixed prosthodontic restorations. Whilst the dentist concerned recognised his shortcomings and accepted responsibility for them in this single case, the GDC were nevertheless concerned about his departure from good practice by not adequately warning of the risks associated with the proposed treatment, not providing a written treatment plan with costings, inadequate clinical planning of the case, poor record keeping and a failure to refer to an appropriately qualified colleague for continuing care. The dentist was not found guilty of serious professional misconduct, but the committee expressed its disapproval of his management.

Example 2

A dentist made 20 claims to the Dental Practice Board for payment to which he knew he was not entitled. In a number of cases, he altered the forms in order to mislead the Dental Practice Board into believing that he was entitled to these payments. In an attempt to defend himself, he fabricated periodontal records for 18 patients. He was found guilty of serious professional misconduct and was erased from the register.

Example 3

A dentist was found not to have explained in advance the treatment he proposed to a patient's tooth, and also failed to obtain consent and explain clearly the costs of the proposed treatment. The dentist also admitted that when treating the patient he did not wear surgical gloves and was not assisted by a dental nurse or other person. As a direct result, the committee believed that he increased the risk of cross infection and compromised his ability to provide cardiopulmonary resuscitation if necessary. He was found guilty of serious professional misconduct and admonished.

has been brought to the GDC's attention) says about that professional's current and future suitability to continue on the register, as part of an overall assessment of their fitness for continuing registration.

---

[i] Anonymised cases taken from the GDC Gazette, Summer 2003–Spring 2004 issues

Example 4

This was a single case where the dentist was advised by a consultant orthodontist to extract some teeth but mistakenly extracted the wrong premolar. Although this case involved only one patient, the committee reached its conclusion because of the combination of factors involved. In addition to his clinical error, the dentist practised without professional indemnity, failed to deal appropriately with the complaint at the time, and failed repeatedly over a long period to respond to letters from the patient's family and their solicitors. The GDC said this fell far below the high standard which the public and the dental profession had a right to expect, and found him guilty of serious professional misconduct and admonished him.

Example 5

The GDC heard evidence in this case about a dentist's clinical knowledge and skills, involving both diagnostic methods and standards of treatment. He had provided restorations which were found to be unnecessary and inappropriate, and which resulted in permanent damage to healthy teeth. No good clinical rationale was advanced for his actions but the committee perceived that they were prompted by non-clinical considerations. There was also evidence of dishonesty in attempting to claim fraudulently from the Dental Practice Board. The dentist was found guilty of serious professional misconduct and erased.

This more holistic approach offers greater flexibility and lends itself to looking at wider issues of professionalism, communication with patients and teamwork skills, as well as the technical 'standards-of-care' aspects that are the common feature of clinical cases.

Fitness to practise

Under the amendment of 2004, the fitness to practise of a registrant may be impaired because of :

- misconduct
- deficient physical performance
- adverse physical or mental health
- a conviction or caution in the UK for a criminal offence, or a conviction elsewhere for an act which if committed in the UK would be an offence
- the ruling of another regulatory body that the registrant's fitness to practise is impaired—this could mean that in the case of a doubly qualified dentist on both the GMC and GDC register, a determination in one will be notified to the other
- an allegation referring to conduct which occurred outside the UK or before the person was registered.

Investigating Committee

Under the amendments envisaged in the section 60 order, an allegation will be referred in most cases to the registrar and then on to the Investigating Committee. This committee does not currently exist, as part of its function is now carried out by the Preliminary Proceeding Committee, which will be replaced.

The registrant will be notified and will be invited to put comments to the Investigating Committee for their consideration. Rules of evidence normally governing legal procedures will be observed in investigating any allegation made against a registrant, and they have two main options available to them. If the committee feels the allegation does not warrant further consideration by one of the fitness to practise committees, it will take no further action. It may also issue a warning to the registrant regarding their future conduct, performance or practice. This may also take the form of advising the registrant that the matter under consideration will remain on file and may be referred to if any further allegations are made of a similar nature.

The Investigating Committee may also reprimand the registrant or offer advice to any other person involved in the investigation or in regard to any issue arising in the course of their investigation.

If the committee decides the allegation should be considered further it can refer the matter to the Health Committee, the Professional Performance Committee, the Professional Conduct Committee or the Interim Orders Committee.

Professional Conduct Committee (PCC)

The Professional Conduct Committee for any particular case will be drawn from the Fitness to Practise Panel. This has 35 panel members (15 dentists, 15 lay members and 5 PCDs). The intention is that where a particular registrant is being investigated, their speciality (e.g. general dental practice, PCD, etc.) will be reflected in the make-up of the PCC for that case. The PCC will investigate the allegations, and under strict rules of evidence will be required to prove each allegation on the criminal standard of proof, i.e. beyond reasonable doubt. The committee will sit with a legal assessor, who is a qualified lawyer and can give advice about the legal process.

The proceedings, open to public and press, are like standard court proceedings where the registrant respondent (the person answering to the complaint) would normally be present throughout and represented by a barrister (counsel-instructed and funded by the registrant's defence organisation), will be cross-examined by a barrister instructed by the GDC who act as the 'prosecutor', and will also have to answer questions from the PCC. Witnesses can be called by both sides.

If the allegations are not proved, the committee is required to publish a statement to that effect, subject to the registrant's consent. If the allegations are proven, the committee (in private) will decide whether the proven facts demonstrate the registrant's fitness to practise is impaired. In that case they can either:

- erase the registrant
- suspend the registrant's registration for up to 12 months
- impose conditions on the registrant's registration for a maximum of 3 years, the continuing registration being therefore conditional on complying with certain requirements, for example not practising unsupervised, not providing certain treatments or to certain categories of patients
- reprimand the registrant.

The PCC has further powers to review cases it has made determinations on and would be free to either remove or extend those original sanctions, depending on the conduct and performance of the registrants in the meantime. The registrant has a right of appeal against any decision made by the GDC through a process called judicial review to the Privy Council, as does the Council for Healthcare Regulatory Excellence (CHRE; see below), who may appeal a decision if they believe the GDC has been unduly lenient.

Any dentist erased will have the opportunity to apply to be restored on to the list before the expiration of the minimum erasure time. At the time of writing, this minimum erasure time is 12 months but the Government is proposing a period of 5 years. Both the GDC and the British Dental Association oppose this on the grounds that such a sanction is more akin to punishment and a disciplinary regime than a system for the protection of the public, and that it could be regarded as unfair and disproportionate. If the period is extended to 5 years, the registrant will only have two attempts in that period of erasure to apply successfully to get back on the list.

Guidance to the Professional Conduct Committee about what action to take if a person's fitness to practise is deemed impaired can be quite illuminating. Erasure is regarded as being merited when certain behaviours are considered so damaging to a registrant's fitness to practise, and to public confidence in the dental profession, that this sanction is the only appropriate outcome. The list given below, whilst not exhaustive or intended to cover all situations, suggests also that not to erase in these situations would require careful justification:

- Serious abuse of the clinical relationship.
- Other serious abuse of the privileged position enjoyed by registered professionals, e.g. prescribing powers, patient trust in terms of 'expert' advice.
- Causing serious avoidable harm to patients deliberately or by reckless substandard care.
- Putting patients in the way of serious avoidable harm by failing to maintain safe standards in relation to premises, equipment and other aspects of the clinical environment—this would include radiation safety and infection control.
- Failure to maintain professional knowledge and competence in areas relevant to the registrant's practice—thus failure to do CPD would result in erasure.
- Violence and unlawful indecent acts.
- Failure to maintain appropriate indemnity or otherwise ensure adequate protection for patients.

Professional Performance Committee

The Professional Performance Committee has the same sanctions open to it that the PCC has, except erasure. There is as yet (because this committee had not come into existence at the time of writing) very little guidance on what matters relating to the registrant's conduct will be brought before the committee.

Health Committee

The Health Committee will be entitled to consider a matter where a registrant's fitness to practise may be impaired by health-related problems. Its method of operation is based in statute and is to be found in a detailed document—*The General Dental Council Health Committee (procedure) Rules Order of Council 1984*.

The committee sits in private and is not open to the press or public. It consists of five people, of whom at least two are registered dentists and at least two are lay persons. Notification to the GDC of a registrant's fitness to practise on grounds of health may come from a colleague or from another GDC committee. The registrant, upon notification of the Health Committee's involvement, will be invited to submit to examination by at least two medical examiners chosen by the GDC. The registrant can obtain an independent medical report.

The medical assessors will be asked to report on the fitness of the dentist to engage in practice, either generally or on limited basis, and on their recommended management of the case. The dentist or a representative will be invited to give oral evidence at a hearing, and witnesses can also be called and examined and cross-examined by both sides.

The Health Committee has the power to suspend the registrant for up to 12 months or impose conditions on continued practice if they judge the fitness-to-practise of the dentist to be seriously impaired by reason of physical or mental condition. In coming to this conclusion, the Committee can take into account the dentist's current or continuing and episodic condition, or a condition which although currently in remission may be expected to cause recurrence of serious impairment.

These cases are often unfortunate tales of drug or drink addiction and inevitably involve a degree of psychiatric impairment, where issues of judgement and rational behaviour are considered. These may also encompass organic psychiatric disorders.

COUNCIL FOR HEALTHCARE REGULATORY EXCELLENCE (CHRE)

One major public concern is the dental profession's ability to deal effectively with its own members. In order to oversee the regulatory functions of the General Dental Council (as well as nine other professional bodies including the General Medical Council, the General Optical Council, the General Osteopathic Council, the General Chiropractic Council, etc.) an overarching body was created—the Council for Healthcare Regulatory Excellence (CHRE).

The Act that brought this body into being was the National Health Service Reform and Healthcare Professions Act 2002 (Part 2, section 25). Originally designated the Council for the Regulation of Healthcare Professionals (CRHP), the body changed its name to the Council for Healthcare Regulatory Excellence in July, 2004. The CHRE is a UK-wide organisation and the Act gives it authority to:

- promote the interests of the public and patients in relation to the regulation of healthcare professions
- promote best practice in the regulation of healthcare professions
- develop principles for good, professionally led regulation of healthcare professions
- promote cooperation between regulators and other organisations.

The CHRE has 19 members—one representative from each of the nine regulators (who is usually the president) and 10 'lay' members.

Its biggest impact on dental practitioners will be on those dentists who find themselves on the receiving end of a sanction from the General Dental Council's Professional Conduct Committee. If the CHRE considers that this sanction has been 'unduly lenient' in respect of a finding of professional misconduct or fitness to practise, or lack of a finding or in regard to any penalty imposed, they can refer the case to the High Court or the Court of Session (in Scotland).

The CHRE has 4 weeks to respond from the date on which the dentist concerned received the decision from the PCC, and therefore the dentist could face the potential stress of yet another hearing if the GDC decision is appealed by the CHRE. The Court of Appeal has recognised that there is an element of double jeopardy, with the dentist being tried twice, but concluded that this was of secondary importance to the need to protect the public.

There is an automatic notice of relevant decisions to the CHRE by the regulators, and in the period September 2003 to October 2004, 526 cases were notified to CHRE for consideration. Of these, only 42 were considered in more detail at case meetings, and 13 cases were referred to the High Court. One of these was from the General Dental Council. This is despite the fact that in the Commons Committee stage of the Bill establishing the CRHP, the Minister said that the need to refer cases to court would be only 'as a last resort to deal with exceptionally grave cases in which there has been a perverse decision or the public interest has not been fully or properly served...we believe that there will be very few cases—perhaps one or two a year'.[4]

NATIONAL CLINICAL ASSESSMENT AUTHORITY (NCAA)

The NCAA was a special health authority that was established in April 2001 following recommendations made in the Chief Medical Officer's reports: 'Supporting doctors, protecting patients'[5] and 'Assuring the quality of medical practice: implementing supporting doctors, protecting patients'[6]. The NCAA provides a service to support the NHS in dealing with doctors and dentists whose performance gives cause for concern. They are able to provide advice to PCTs and Trusts about the local handling of cases, and where necessary carry out clinical performance assessments to clarify areas of concern and make recommendations on how difficulties may be resolved.

In order to help doctors and dentists in difficulty, the NCAA provides advice, takes referrals and carries out targeted assessments where necessary. The NCAA's assessment involves trained medical and lay assessors. This is a full clinical performance assessment of the dentist, which considers clinical capability, health, behaviour and job context.

Once an objective assessment has been carried out, the NCAA will advise on the appropriate course of action. The NCAA does not take over the role of an employer, nor does it function as a regulator. The NCAA is established as an advisory body, and the NHS employer organisation remains responsible for resolving the problem once the NCAA has produced its assessment. As part of the development of systems and processes, the NCAA has liaised with regulatory and investigatory bodies such as the General Medical Council (GMC), Commission for Health Improvement (CHI) and the National Patient Safety Agency (NPSA), with whom it has developed memoranda of understanding. These are designed to ensure easy and swift cooperation, recognise each other's distinct areas of operation and allow for fast-track referral of cases between the organisations to ensure that cases are responded to by the appropriate body.

As part of the DoH's review of its arm's length bodies in June 2004, the NCAA was brought together with the National Patient Safety Agency (NPSA), and established as a separate, self-contained division within the new agency, known as the National Clinical Assessment Service (NCAS).

The authority also conducts research and development into how performance problems can be identified and addressed, and runs an external education programme to support NHS managers in dealing with performance issues.

PATIENT COMPLAINTS IN DENTAL PRACTICE

A dissatisfied patient in general dental practice has a number of options open to them. They can simply vote with their feet and find themselves another practice. They may wish to complain to the practice themselves, or the health authority if the complaint is to do with the provision of services under an NHS contract. Or they may complain to the General Dental Council.

This section gives a broad outline of the three stages of the NHS system of complaints. It then goes on to describe briefly what happens at the GDC if a patient writes directly to complain about a dentist. This may be the only avenue open to them if treatment was carried out under private contract. Some general practitioners treat patients either under an insurance type scheme such as Denplan or as part of a quality assurance scheme such as the BDA Good Practice Scheme. Both these schemes have procedures in operation if a patient should make a complaint about the services they have received.

From the introduction of the National Health Service in 1948 up until 1990, there was no official separate procedure for complaints, and these were dealt with under the service committee procedures as set out in the regulations. Thus, complaints and discipline cases were inextricably linked, to the detriment of both patients and practitioners.

Fundamental to the progress of the complaint was the identification of a breach of one or more of the practitioner's Terms of Service. Without this, there was no complaint to answer and the patient was left with no further options under the NHS.

Pre-1996: the 'old system'

Criticism of the NHS complaints system in the 1980s and 1990s centred on three issues: a) it was biased towards dentists, b) the procedures were opaque and c) it focussed too much on disciplining rather than resolution of the patient's complaint. In 1993, in response to the disquiet amongst professionals, academics and patient interest groups, the Wilson Committee was asked by the Government to review the NHS complaints procedure. They reported their findings in 'Being heard—the report of the committee on NHS complaints procedures' (1994).[7] The committee identified nine principles that should be introduced into any NHS complaints procedure: responsiveness, quality enhancement, cost effectiveness, accessibility, impartiality, simplicity, speed, confidentiality and accountability.

Their conclusions ran to over 60 recommendations but fundamental was:

- introduction of a single procedure applicable throughout the NHS
- a three-stage process involving 'local resolution', 'independent review' and the Health Service Commissioner (HSC)
- an extension of the HSC's jurisdiction to GDPs (and other Part II practitioners) so as to cover 'clinical judgement' complaints.[8]

The government accepted the Wilson Committee's recommendations in 'Acting on complaints' in March 1995, and on April 1, 1996 the 'new complaints' procedure was introduced

into the NHS for doctors and dentists. The most significant change was the separation of the complaints procedure from disciplinary procedures, thus allowing a wider range of issues to be addressed within the complaints procedure. It also meant that practitioners would be more likely to engage fully with the process knowing that disciplinary issues were not the usual endpoint to the investigations.

Post-1996: the 'new system' and future reforms of the complaints system

For dentists, the need to have a practice-based complaints procedure and to publicise it became an NHS Terms of Service requirement.

(1) Subject to sub-paragraph (2) a dentist shall establish, and operate in accordance with this paragraph, a procedure (in this paragraph and in paragraph 31B referred to as a 'practice based complaints procedure') to deal with any complaints made by or on behalf of his patients and former patients.

In terms of scope, the complaints procedure applies:

…to complaints made in relation to any matter reasonably connected with the dentist's provision of general dental services and within the responsibility or control of
a) the dentist
b) any other dentist either employed by him or engaged as a deputy
c) a former partner of the dentist
d) any employee of the dentist other than one falling within paragraph (b)

The paragraph goes on to outline who should be responsible for receiving and investigating complaints, who can make a complaint, the time limits for an acknowledgement (3 days) and full response (10 days), and the need to inform patients about the existence of the complaints procedure and the named complaints manager.[9]

There is a further requirement to provide the health authority with an annual return, specifying the number of complaints received by the practice where all other dentists are included on the dental list and are working together.[10]

In addition to there being a terms of service requirement for NHS practitioners, the GDC expects that 'if a patient has cause to complain about the service provided, every effort should be made to resolve the matter at practice level' and that the Council 'endorses the detailed guidance on handling complaints which has been issued by the NHS Executive and the British Dental Association and would expect compliance'[11]

The details of the current complaints procedure are to be found in the NHS Executive document: *Complaints: listening, acting, improving: guidance pack for general dental practitioners (1996)*.[12]

Complaints manager

The intention of having a complaints manager is to ensure one person has an overview of the whole complaints system and will assume the task of coordinating the correspondence and replies. The person nominated to administer the complaints procedure should be identified as such to patients. In a small practice it is usually the dentist who acts as the complaints manager, but this would be inappropriate if the complaint was about that particular dentist. In this case another member of staff should act as the coordinator.

Complaints and disciplinary procedures to be separated

> *4.28 Policy remains firm on the need for the new complaints procedure to be concerned only with resolving complaints and not with investigating disciplinary matters. The purpose of the complaints procedure is not to apportion blame amongst staff. It is to investigate complaints with the aim of satisfying the complainant (while being scrupulously fair to staff) and to learn any lessons for improvement in service delivery.*[13]

Because of the previous intertwining of the complaints procedure with discipline, unless the complaint could be framed in such a way as to fall within a dentist's terms of service, it could not be considered. The aim of separation was therefore to widen the scope of the complaints procedure but at the same time remove the threat of disciplinary action from the dentist.

Information gathered in the complaints process by the practitioner as part of local resolution, belongs to the practice and is kept separate from the patient's records. The Health

Authority therefore has no right of access to it and, it could be argued, neither does the patient. It was felt by the Wilson committee that this guidance was necessary to avoid repercussions for the patient later if it is known they have made a complaint about the practice in the past, especially as the notes will be transferred on to any new doctor who sees the patient. In the case of general dental practice the notes remain with the practice and are seldom transferred to other practices.

A practitioner must consent to its release and it cannot be made available automatically for use in disciplinary investigations, although the Ombudsman has powers to require the production of information and documents.[14]

Possible claims for negligence[15]

> *4.37 The complaints procedure should cease if the complainant explicitly indicates an intention to take legal action in respect of a complaint.*

The guidance in relation to this issue makes it clear that responding to the complaint openly may be sufficient to satisfy the complainant, even if the initial contact is via a solicitor's letter. The reality is that communication has already broken down between the patients and dentist, and it would be hard to reconcile differences through the mediation of a 'no win no fee' solicitor. A dentist would be unwise to make admissions in these circumstances despite the guidance that 'a hostile, or defensive, reaction to the complaint is more likely to encourage the complainant to seek information and a remedy through the courts' (para 4.38).

> *4.39 In all prima facie cases of negligence, or where the complainant has indicated the intention to start legal proceedings, the principles of good claims management and risk management should be applied. There should be a full and thorough investigation of the events.*

Where it is appropriate, defence organisations may advise a dentist to settle the matter by a reimbursement of fees or an *ex gratia* payment.

Local resolution—stage one

Local resolution is the first part of a three-stage process that is common to all sectors of the NHS.

The intention is to make this part of the process responsive enough to deal with the majority of the complaints received by a general dental practitioner, the aim being that the practice itself deals with the problem quickly and efficiently.

A complaint can come either verbally, in person or on the phone, or in writing. It may be directed to the practice or to the heath authority. In the latter case, the health authority advises in the first instance that the complainant writes or contacts the dental practice concerned to make their complaint. Complaints may be made about virtually any aspect of healthcare and are not confined to the treatment provided.

The response times for general practices are expected to be an acknowledgement within two days and a full response within ten working days.[16] These are for guidance only but it is generally accepted that the longer the delay in responding, the more entrenched both parties may become. However, staff may be on holiday, have moved to another practice or are awaiting advice and draft letters from their defence organisations and therefore these guidelines are often overlooked.

Conciliation

As part of the local resolution stage, conciliation should be offered where, following an investigation, an immediate oral response seems inappropriate or where the complainant remains dissatisfied following an earlier response. The health authority may already have become involved if the complainant has written directly to them. In this case the health authority normally writes to the dentist, enclosing a copy of the complaint with an offer to use the services of their lay conciliator. This is provided free of charge to both parties, but both parties need to agree to it.

Conciliation is used when a person wishes to complain under a practice-based procedure, and it would (in the opinion of the health authority) be unreasonable to expect the complaint to be made directly to the dentist concerned, or where the complainant is dissatisfied with the investigation carried out in the practice-based procedure.[17]

The complainant should be advised of the complaints procedure and that they have a right to seek an independent review if they remain unhappy with the practice-based response.

Independent review—stage two

Complainants who are not happy with the practice-based response may seek an independent review of the matter. They may do this only in relation to NHS services. Where private dental treatment has been provided, and that is the source of complaint, they do not normally have access to this system.

Up until 2004, the independent review stage was carried out by the health authority who, via a screener, reviewed the complainant's request to establish an Independent Review Panel (IRP). There was no absolute right to an independent review, and it was a matter for the convenor's discretion. This stage (most of all) was criticised as lacking any real independence, and the decision-making process by the panels was inconsistent, primarily because they sat so infrequently.

In response to these and other concerns, the 1996 complaints procedure underwent an independent evaluation during 1999–2000. The evaluation report (NHS complaints procedure national evaluation) and a listening document (Reforming the NHS complaints procedure—a listening document) were published in 2001. In 2003, the Department of Health published NHS complaints reform—making things right, which described proposals to reform the NHS complaints procedure. This resulted in further legislative changes and came into force in July 2004 as the 'National Health Service (Complaints) Regulations 2004'. These regulations do not cover the local resolution stage of complaints in general dental practice, as these remain regulated by The National Health Service (General Dental Services) Amendment Regulations 1996.

The original intention was to implement the reformed complaints in procedure in full from June 2004, but Ministers decided to phase it in after the 5th report from the Shipman Inquiry, which published in December 2004. The reports from the Neale and Ayling inquiries will also influence the direction of the complaints procedures.

The new arrangements do apply to general dental practitioners for independent review, as set out in part III of the complaints regulations.

Healthcare Commission

The Healthcare Commission (formerly known as the Commission for Healthcare Audit and

Inspection) took over the second stage of the NHS procedure in England and Wales in July 2004. They cannot consider a complaint where the complainant has stated in writing an intention to take legal proceedings.

All requests for an independent review will be acknowledged within two days. The requests to involve the Healthcare Commission can come from the patient, or trusts with the patient's consent. There will then be an initial review during which a member of the Healthcare Commissioners Complaints Team will review the case, with the help of expert advice if necessary, to determine whether further investigation is needed. A letter with the decision and any recommendations will be sent to the complainant and the practitioner about whom the complaint is made, within 20 days. The Healthcare Commission at this point can refer the complainant to the GDC or the Health Service Commissioner.

If the Healthcare Commission decides to carry out a further investigation itself, the terms of reference will be sent to the complainant and the practitioner they are complaining about for comment, and both parties will receive a full report of their findings at the end of the investigation. The Healthcare Commission has wide discretion to conduct its investigation in any manner it sees fit and may take any advice it deems to be required.

If the complainant is unhappy with the outcome of the investigation, they have a right to request an independent panel to hear their concerns. The panel will consist of three members of the panel who are unconnected to the NHS but are trained in dealing with complaints. The panel will hear from both sides of the complaint, and a participant before a panel may be accompanied or represented by a friend or advocate but not by a legal representative acting as such. The panel will then make recommendations for resolution and/or for improving the services where appropriate.

Health Service Commissioner (Ombudsman) (HSC)—stage three

The Health Service Ombudsman is the third tier of the complaints system in the NHS. The Health Service Commissioners for England and Wales came into existence as a result of the National Health Service Reorganisation Act 1973 (subsequently Part V of the National Health Service Act

1977) but their jurisdiction is now defined by the Health Service Commissioners Act 1993 (as amended).

In accepting the recommendations from the Wilson Committee, the government extended the jurisdiction of the Health Service Commissioners to complaints against dentists (and other Part II practitioners) and to those involving clinical judgement in section 6 of the Health Service Commissioners (Amendment) Act 1996. This was a new step but recognised by the Health Service Commissioner at the time, William Reid, as being another burden: 'I well understand the concern of professionals about the potential multiple jeopardy they face—from the courts, the regulatory bodies and now the Ombudsman—when encountering complaints about their practice'.[18]

The HSC can only investigate a dentist where it has received a complaint by or on behalf of a person if they have sustained injustice or hardship in consequence of action taken by the family health service provider. Action includes inaction and a failure to provide a service.[19]

Any complaint about a dentist to the HSC must be about action related to NHS services the provider has undertaken to deliver. This means that dental treatment provided under private contract falls outside the remit of the HSC, although there have been investigations conducted where the patient *believed* they were having NHS treatment when in fact it was private. The HSC can also investigate, amongst other bodies: health authorities, primary care trusts and the Dental Practice Board.

Before the HSC can investigate a complaint, it must be demonstrated that the complainant pursued the matter under the local resolution phase. An investigation cannot be instigated until those procedures have been 'invoked and exhausted', unless in the particular circumstance of a case it is reasonable for this to happen.

There are statutory limits to what can be investigated by the HSC. These include complaints about personnel issues, actions taken by health authorities in connection with disciplinary cases (the old service committees) and commercial or contractual matters.

Legal remedy

The HSC cannot investigate complaints about matters where the complainant has or had:

- a right of appeal, reference or review to or before a tribunal constituted by or under any enactment or by virtue of Her Majesty's prerogative
- a remedy by way of proceedings in any court.[20]

In this context, the professional regulatory bodies, such as the General Dental Council, are not regarded as tribunals. The legislation allows the Ombudsman to investigate complaints of this kind only if satisfied that in the particular circumstances it is not reasonable to expect the complainant to resort to legal remedy; but the Ombudsman cannot investigate if the complainant has gone to court.

Time limits

The Commissioner shall not entertain the complaint if it is made more than a year after the day on which the person aggrieved first had notice of the matters alleged in complaint, unless he considers it reasonable to do so.[21] These time limits differ from the three year limit imposed by the Limitation Act, and it can be argued from the patient's perspective, the desire to protect staff from the fear of complaints is surely not good enough reason for imposing a time limit of a single year.[22]

All complaints are screened to establish whether they fall within the remit of the HSC and whether there is a practical reason to investigate (i.e. will achieve something). It is entirely at the HSC discretion whether to investigate or not.

A Statement of complaint, setting out the 'terms of reference', is sent to the dentist and they are invited to submit comments. These comments are important in the work of the HSC. As part of the investigation the dentist and the patient(s) will be interviewed (separately). An assessor may also produce a report when clinical matters are considered.

Remedy

The HSC does not have the power to award compensation, but they can recommend *ex-gratia* payments to cover out-of-pocket expenses. HSC can and often does ask for an apology to be made in the report, and can also ask that a review of the procedures take place in the practice.

The HSC also has the power to disclose information about any person discovered in the course of an investigation to the General Dental Council if considered necessary in the interests of the protection of the health and safety of patients. In such cases, the Ombudsman must inform the individual about whom the information has been passed.

Complaints to the General Dental Council

Patients who feel aggrieved about the service they have received from a dental practitioner often copy their letter of complaint to the General Dental Council. They do this either because they feel the practitioner will be forced to respond to the complaint rather than ignore it, or they genuinely feel the dentist should be prevented from practising.

The NHS complaints system is well established and easily accessible to patients. An increasing number of dental patients in the UK are being treated either wholly or partially under private contract.

As described above, a patient is able to make a complaint directly to the General Dental Council. If the patient has had private treatment there will be a Private Patients Complaint Scheme, which is intended to mirror the NHS scheme in terms of having a local resolution element to it and a second stage external review of the complaint.

First stage

The first stage of this scheme will provide an information service, including a telephone helpline which will be open to anyone who has a query about their dental treatment. NHS complaints will be referred to the appropriate NHS authority, and the patients will be encouraged to try and settle the problem directly with the practice concerned.

It is sometimes difficult to separate NHS from private complaints entirely. The patients may indeed be complaining about that very issue, where they believe they were receiving NHS care when in fact they were charged under a private contract. Sometimes the treatment may have been carried out under private contract on an NHS patient but the complaint relates to other issues, such as infection control.

Second stage

If the complaint is not resolved by the practice, the scheme will act as an intermediary between the patient and the practice to try and help resolve the complaint. A panel may be convened and will make recommendations about how the complaint should be resolved. If at any stage the panel believes the conduct of the registrants concerned gives rise for wider concerns, they can refer the matter to the Investigating Committee of the GDC.

FURTHER READING

Harris J. The value of life: an introduction to medical ethics. London: Routledge; 1997.

Hope T, Savulescu J, Hendrick J. Medical ethics and law: the core curriculum. Edinburgh: Churchill Livingstone; 2003.

Martin J. The English Legal System. 3rd edn. London: Hodder and Stoughton; 2002.

NCAA Handbook. Autumn 2004 (www.ncaaa.nhs.uk)

REFERENCES

1 Kennedy I, Grubb A. Medical Law. 3rd edn. London: Butterworths; 2000.
2 Beauchamp TL, Childress JF. Principles of biomedical ethics. 5th edn. New York: Oxford University Press; 2001.
3 Learning from Bristol: the report of the public enquiry into children's heart surgery at the Bristol Royal Infirmary 1984–1995. The Stationery Office; 2001.
4 Hansard House of Commons Standing Committee A, 13 December 2001, 9 cols 424–427.
5 Supporting Doctors, Protecting Patients: a consultation paper on preventing, recognising and dealing with poor performance in doctors in the NHS in England. National Health Service; 1999.
6 Assuring the quality of medical practice: implementing supporting doctors, protecting patients. Department of Health; 2001.
7 Being heard—the report of the committee on NHS complaints procedures. Department of Health; 1994.
8 Kennedy I, Grubb A. Medical Law. 3rd edn. London: Butterworths; 2000.
9 National Health Service (General Dental Services) Regulations 1992, Sch 1, Part IV, para 31A.
10 Ibid., para 31C.
11 Maintaining standards. General Dental Council. Para 3.13.
12 Complaints, acting, improving: guidance on the implementation of the NHS Complaints Procedure. NHS Executive; 1996.
13 Ibid., para 4.28.
14 Ibid., para 4.31.
15 Ibid., para 4.37–4.39.
16 Ibid., para 5.14.
17 Directions to health authorities on dealing with complaints about family health service practitioners. National Health Service in England and Wales; 1996: art 12.
18 Reid W. Introduction. In: A guide to the work of the Health Service Ombudsman. Office of the Health Service Commissioner for England; 1996.
19 Health Service Commissioners Act 1993 (as amended), section 3(1).
20 Ibid., section 4(1).
21 Ibid., section 8(4).
22 Harpwood V. The Health Service Commissioner: the extended role in the new NHS. European Journal of Law 1996; 3:207.

Off the record

2

Clinical dental records are primarily designed to record treatment carried out on a patient, and they act as an historical record. They are essential to the delivery of dental care, contributing to the processes of diagnosis, treatment planning and the provision of care in an ordered manner. Clinical records are a communication tool, allowing a patient's care to be accessed by the treating dentist, the patient themselves and other healthcare workers.

They assume an important significance when a patient either complains or makes a claim in negligence, or something goes wrong. One of the most frustrating aspects of analysing dental notes is discovering that a dentist's legal position is undermined by the lack of supportive information in the patient's clinical records, even when the treatment provided has been of a high standard.

Record keeping is often considered an afterthought by practitioners, used merely to record treatment items, to note financial or administrative functions, and often not much else. The rise of consumerism means that patients' expectations of their care is higher, and patients are ever more ready to question the care they have been given. Threat of litigation has prompted many dentists to change their note taking procedures and improve the explanations given to patients.[1]

Therefore, records will come under increasing scrutiny of patients, their legal advocates, statutory NHS bodies, third party payers and regulatory bodies such as the General Dental Council. Poor record keeping can make it difficult or impossible to defend claims of clinical negligence or professional misconduct. It can lead to disputes over money and can cost a practice large sums, and can even have the most serious (and fatal) consequences.

WHAT ARE RECORDS?

A medical record is any record which contains information relating to the physical or mental health or condition of an individual and has been made by or on behalf of a medical professional in connection with the treatment of that individual.[i] In this context, dental records can therefore cover a wide range of material (Box 2.1).

STANDARDS IN RECORD KEEPING

Whilst there is no standard data set for dental records, there are some key elements common to all good records. The first and most important of these is that the records are contemporaneous— that is, 'recorded at the time'. Entries should be dated, summarising the treatment provided for the patient, including what the patient reports to you, and results of any investigations, such as pulp testing, percussion and pain history. The

---

Box 2.1 What do records comprise?

- Handwritten clinical notes (record cards/envelopes) including medical history
- Computerised records
- X-ray films and other imaging records (and tracings if relevant)
- Investigations (pathology reports, printouts from monitoring equipment)
- Models
- Photographs
- Correspondence between health professionals
- Other information, e.g. laboratory instructions and receipts, estimates
- Videos
- Tape recordings of telephone conversations

---

[i] Definition from the Health Professions Council

second requirement is the completion in writing of a medical history by the patient, or parent if a child. There are many types of pro forma for this, and each patient is expected to complete one at the initial visit. This should be subsequently updated with any changes noted. If the medical history remains unchanged, this should also be noted.

Computer records, with the potential for using custom screens, function keys with set texts and detailed printed patient estimates, can be extremely useful. They can, unfortunately, also be used simply to record treatment codes or tooth notation, and nothing else.

Excellent records will help the dentist and others to understand not only what was done, when and how, but more importantly to appreciate why it was done—the thought processes and logic behind the actions. They will capture details that could be pivotal to the final outcome if a complaint or claim is ever raised (Box 2.2 and Table 2.1).

ORAL HEALTH SCORES

Healthcare provision is moving to outcome measures as a way of judging whether dental care has improved over a period of time. Considerable money is spent on dentistry in the UK. The most recent estimate from the Office of Fair Trading puts it at £3.8 billion in 2003–04, with the private sector making up £1.9 billion of this figure. It is estimated that private sector treatment will increase by 47% between 2003 and 2007.

The Oral Health Index was developed by Burke and Wilson in the mid-1990's.[2] It covers aspects of the patient's satisfaction with his or her mouth, assessment of caries, the restorations, wear, periodontal condition, occlusion and dentures. This is a reproducible score, and it is an easy way to provide the practitioner with a means of measuring the effectiveness of treatment and improving communication with patients.[3]

BASELINE CHARTING

It is important that all patients have a baseline charting done of all existing restorations. This establishes the basis upon which future treatment is carried out, but it is also useful in the event of the need to forensically identify the patient. Dental identification was the prime method of identifying the victims of the 9/11 terrorist attack in New York and Washington, as well as the tsunami earthquake disaster in Indonesia and the surrounding countries in December 2004.

Forensic dental identification uses ante-mortem records, such as dental chartings, radiographs and photographs taken by general dental practitioners, to compare with post mortem records taken by forensic odontologists on-site at the scene. In an era where increasing numbers of patients have few or no restorations, other identifying features such as a midline diastema, rotated teeth and tori can usefully be recorded in the notes for future reference. One study concluded that the two major problems that have faced forensic odontologists for decades are the failure by dental practitioners throughout the world to maintain comprehensive records, particularly full-mouth chartings and the failure to add patient names to dentures.[4]

BATCH NUMBERS

For completeness, the batch numbers of any drugs used on or by patients should be recorded. There is no absolute legal requirement to do so (e.g. for local anaesthetic administration), but it may be prudent to do so where a patient has an allergic reaction or side-effect immediately following an injection. This may be useful if product liability needs to be established under the Consumer Protection Act 1987.

Box 2.2 What should a written record contain?

- Up-to-date medical history
- The date, diagnosis and treatment notes every time the patient is seen, with full details of any particular incidents, episodes or discussions including options
- Monitoring information such as BPE scores, periodontal probing depths and other indices, tracking oral pathology and other conditions
- All payments made by the patient
- All correspondence to and from the patient, or any third party (consultant, other dentists, doctor, etc)
- Consents obtained and warnings and information given
- Findings/diagnosis on radiographs—particularly if discovered after the patient has left the surgery
- Drugs and dosages given

Table 2.1 Ten essential requirements in clinical record keeping

Identification data	These will include name, address, telephone numbers and e-mail addresses. Text messages (SMS, short message service) are being increasingly used by practices to remind patients of appointments and so mobile phone numbers are useful
Medical history	This should be in the form of a written pro forma which will cover all aspects of the patient's general health. This should be signed and dated by the patient and have a space for the treating dentist to date every time the medical history is checked at recalls. There should be an enquiry about smoking and alcohol consumption
Dental history	This should cover previous dental experiences, why the patient has come to the particular practice, as well as an understanding of risk factors such as diet, and oral hygiene measures. Lifestyle questions about attitudes to dentistry and cosmetic treatment can be covered in a questionnaire
Clinical examination	This clinical examination should cover both extra-oral as well as intra-oral structures, including an oral cancer screening. Both negative and positive findings should be recorded. A baseline charting to include the current status of the teeth and supporting periodontal structures should be undertaken with a record that this has been done. A basic periodontal examination (BPE) or some other equivalent objective measurement should be recorded
Radiographic examination	Any radiographs taken should be justified and the report on any findings should be in the notes
Diagnosis	Very few notes record a diagnosis, except for the most common pericoronitis. A diagnosis gives a rationale for treatment and should be present even for routine fillings, e.g. 'recurrent caries–broken filling' or 'irreversible pulpitis'
Treatment plan	A list of treatment to be done as well as any referral that needs to be made should be recorded. This allows the proper sequencing of treatment according to appropriate principles of relief of pain first, followed by increasingly complex treatment depending on the patient's response to prevention and other advice
Reference to consent	The options available should be discussed and recorded, as well as the relevant advantages and disadvantages. The patient's preference for a particular treatment should be recorded and the reasons for doing so especially if the dentist is not in complete agreement
Progress notes	These will form the bulk of the records and should always be dated and a note made of the treating dentist. The nurse's initials are useful also. The treatments undertaken, details of local anaesthetics and any instructions given should be noted. Some warnings may be given as standard, and to avoid continually recording them, an advice sheet can be given and a copy retained in the file for future reference. These may be on post-extraction instruction, advice about orthodontic appliances or the care of dentures
Exit notes	If a patient informs the practice that they are leaving, it is useful to record the reasons for the departure. This is particularly so if they are in the middle of treatment. Many practices send questionnaires to patients who have not visited the practice for some time and these will assist in developing a customer-orientated approach to patient care. Some patients may request copies of their notes or radiographs when they leave and they are entitled to copies of them under the Data Protection Act

Based on: Rattan R, Tiernan J. Risk Management in General Dental Practice. London: Quintessence; 2004: 95.

ALLERGIES

Allergies in dentistry are becoming an increasing problem. The most common is a type I latex allergy, which is more problematic to clinical staff than patients[5] due to the likely sensitisation to the latex proteins found in natural rubber latex (NRL) gloves over a period of time. Irritant contact dermatitis and type IV reactions are due to the residual chemical employed during the manufacture and processing of medical gloves. A medical history questionnaire will enquire about allergies, and if patients disclose an allergy of this nature it is important to prominently record this in the notes for future reference. The use of latex gloves and rubber dam would be contraindicated in these patients, but there are non-latex alternatives.

Nickel sensitivity is also a problem, and it is important to know what metals the dental laboratories are using to construct the crowns and dental appliances used in patients. Suppliers, aware of this, provide metal content cards, which can be affixed to record cards or kept in the notes. Supplying low cost alloys or non-precious metal crowns may be fraudulent if paid for by the NHS and charged as though they were higher cost alloys. This practice may also be a breach of statute law under the Sale of Goods Act, or breach of contract if a patient specifically asked and paid for a certain content of precious metal in a restoration. A chair-side test is available to sample crowns in a non-invasive manner, and the analysis of the sample can be provided off-site in a laboratory.[6]

GENERAL DENTAL COUNCIL

Standards for Dental Professionals[7] is the General Dental Council guidance on what is to be expected of dentists. Record keeping is highlighted, and the contemporaneous nature of records is also highlighted. Whilst failure to comply strictly with these guidelines with regard to record keeping will not in itself render a dentist liable to a charge of serious professional misconduct, fraudulent record keeping or alterations certainly would.

> Paragraph 1.4
> *Make and keep accurate, complete and contemporaneous patient records including a medical history. Make sure that patients have easy access to their records.*

Maintaining Standards, the previous guidance issued to registrants, was more expansive in detail about record keeping, but the intention behind *Standards for Dental Professionals* is that it should not produce technical guidance or be a rule book.

A number of cases that have come before the Professional Conduct Committee have highlighted poor record keeping as either a contributory factor to the main problem complained of or an important and relevant issue, proven as fact, but not germane to the outcome of the case itself. They have admonished dentists for reconstituting dental records in an inappropriate attempt to overcome administrative problems, for fabrication of dental records, deliberately withholding dental records from patients and keeping poor records that were liable to prejudice future treatment of patients.

NATIONAL HEALTH SERVICE

General dental practitioners holding contract numbers and providing NHS dental treatment are bound by statute regulations (National Health Service Act 1977 [as amended]), which gives rise to secondary legislation—NHS (General Dental Services) Regulations 1992. These regulations establish practitioners' 'terms of service'. These currently make provisions for the requirement of NHS dentists to keep full, accurate and contemporaneous records in respect of the care and treatment given to each patient (Paragraph 25). They also oblige the dentist to retain the records, radiographs and study models for two years after the completion of any course of treatment.

The transition to local commissioning of dental services in England as a result of the National Health Service (Primary Care) Act 1997 has meant more local service level agreements between primary care trusts and dentists, which has resulted in a variety of different contracts and obligations throughout the country.

The changes outlined in the Health and Social Care Act 2003 will also continue to impact on the rights and responsibilities of commissioning agencies and dentists with regard to record keeping, their access by relevant bodies and the need to maintain them.

STATUTE LAW

The Care Standards Act 2000 is quite far reaching, with regulations laying down national minimum standards for, amongst other things, the independent health sector. There are some standards expected in terms of records and information management. It is important that providers are required to have in place written policies and procedures in respect of all records, record keeping and the control of documents.

HOW GOOD IS OUR RECORD KEEPING?

Audit and clinical governance

It is a fact of the human condition that we are always likely to believe our own clinical notes are better than they actually are, and it is clinical audit that settles the matter once and for all.

Clinical audit is defined as the systematic critical analysis of the quality of dental care, including the procedures and processes used for diagnosis, intervention and treatment, the use of resources and the resulting outcome and quality of life as assessed by both professionals and patients.[8]

Clinical audit is an integral part of clinical governance processes in practice and is an essential tool in assuring and improving quality.

The main components of clinical governance are:
- clear lines of responsibility and accountability for the overall quality of clinical care
- a comprehensive programme of quality improvement systems (including clinical audit, supporting and applying evidence based practice, implementing clinical standards and guidelines, workforce planning and development)
- clear policies aimed at managing risk
- procedures for all professional groups to identify and remedy poor performance
- a partnership with patients in the designing and delivery of services.[9]

Total quality management (TQM) techniques, such as ISO 9000, concentrate on administrative procedures to assure quality outcomes. Here the focus is on developing protocols and systems to try and develop a consistent approach to the delivery of healthcare, since in risk management terms this reduces the chances of errors or adverse events.

Good records do not necessarily assure the quality of treatment provided, but they do demonstrate a methodical approach to patient care that is of great benefit if a patient complains or makes a claim in negligence. Record cards are the only instrument capable of documenting all aspects of patient care that can readily be used to gain insight into not only the clinician's adequacy in diagnosis and treatment planning, but also into the sequencing of treatment procedures, their delivery, and in conjunction with radiographs, the technical quality of the procedures themselves.[10]

With hand-written records, legibility is a significant problem. One audit concluded that some dentists could not read their own notes: 'more accurate, understandable reporting could be produced by dictation to the dental assistant, provided that the record is signed by the dentist to ensure its accuracy'.[11]

Records can be audited in such a way as to produce a numerical score. By attributing a numerical score to the assessment, comparisons can be made between the standard of note keeping between individual dentists, between practices and between different specialities or places of work (i.e. hospital, community or general practice setting). The CRABel score has done this quite successfully in auditing medical records in a hospital setting and can be adapted for use in practice to cover the required areas as outlined above.[12]

Abbreviations

Individual dentists often have their own shorthand way of writing up their notes, but this (along with poor handwriting) is one of the biggest areas of confusion in manual records. Computer records do also suffer from codes and abbreviations which may be totally alien to another practitioner or indeed the dentist themselves some time afterwards. As part of clinical governance procedures, any practice abbreviations or note-taking short cuts should be recorded separately and periodically updated. This is also a useful training document for new staff.

Acronyms abound in dentistry and used to be a source of mild amusement between practitioners, especially hospital-based ones. They no longer have any place in records that are open to scrutiny from patients via the Data Protection Act. Trying to explain the following acronyms may be embarrassing:

UBI—unexplained beer injury
GLM—good looking mum
FLK—funny looking kid
DEBA—don't ever book again
PLM—proper little madam
TEETH—tried everything else, try homeopathy
LOBNH—lights on but nobody home
DBI (dirt bag index)—multiplies the number of tattoos with the number of missing teeth to give an estimate of the number of days since the patient last washed: a dental index that has no international recognition or standardisation!

Computerised records

Increasing numbers of practices are moving to computer-based records both for clinical record keeping as well as appointment scheduling. There are many advantages to this from an efficiency perspective, but dento-legal issues are equally important.

Manual records that are currently stored within a card or envelope, such as laboratory sheets, signed medical history forms, credit card slips and correspondence, and details of materials used in a case (e.g. implants and crown metal contents), may be lost in a paper-free practice unless they are scanned and retained electronically. Any of these items may be crucial in the context of a specific investigation about an episode of treatment for a particular patient.

There must be a robust audit trail to any software programme so that any deletions or alterations can easily be identified and retrievable from the hard disc by the supplier if necessary. This has the benefit of demonstrating that any notes recorded were made contemporaneously but equally should deter practitioners from embellishing, altering, deleting or otherwise interfering with the integrity of the records as they existed at the time the original treatment was provided.

Data protection and security are important considerations since access to confidential information should be limited to only those authorised to see it. Entry should be password protected, and users should keep these secure. Many software packages have access to managerial and administration functions, which also need to be password protected so that access to sensitive financial information is restricted.[13]

Carrying out audits of clinical records

Taking as a starting point what should be in a clinical record (Box 2.2 above), it is relatively straightforward to carry out an audit of clinical records in practice. Having first identified the record component, it is important to describe the standard expected. Some of the standards may be legal requirements, whilst others may be 'peer' standards from guidelines which may not have an evidence base but are considered 'good practice'. Many of the guidelines in record keeping are of this nature since there is very little in the way of published evidence that the achievement of certain standards in record keeping delivers a specific quality outcome. See Appendix 2 for an audit template on checking for completeness of records.

One particular audit considered the broad record components of:

- written medical history questionnaire
- examination of soft tissue
- full tooth charting
- periodontal screening and examination
- written diagnosis
- treatment plan.

It concluded that the quality of record keeping was poor, although this was in line with the findings of other worldwide studies. Fundamental clinical entries that could impact on basic dental care provision, such as periodontal screening, were missing from many records.[14]

This study also found that the frequency of recording for patients whose treatment was funded under NHS regulations was significantly worse than for patients whose treatment was privately funded. The reason postulated by the audited dentist in this study was that the time constraints produced by the need to deliver care as quickly as possible under NHS regulations leave little time for accurate record keeping.

A similar level of poor record keeping was found in Sweden. In nearly 40% of the variables investigated, the documentation did not follow the rules and guidelines expected. Patient history, status, diagnosis, therapy plans and other important information were missing from the records of general dental practitioners. However, the specialist records were in general very accurate. Interestingly, dentist age related to the quality of the records, with older practitioners not having as accurate records as younger dentists.[15]

Even before dentists enter practice, their record keeping has been found to be far from optimal. In a study of final year students, even after they had been re-audited, the scores for updated medical history and the patient's complaint had deteriorated.[16] A similar finding emerged amongst dental students in the School of Dentistry in the University of Washington, Seattle.[17]

Membership of the Faculty of General Dental Practitioners (MFGDP) Exam

The MFGDP, which is an entry point to a career pathway in general dental practice, has a number of components to its examination. One of these is the coursework module, which has three units:

- evidence-based portfolio of seven key skills
- audit project
- case report.

The key skills portfolio is based on evidence accumulated from the candidate's practice to demonstrate their understanding of the various principles and standards, and their application in the candidate's own particular practice set up.

These key clinical skills are:

1. prevention and management of medical emergencies in general dental practice
2. cross-infection control
3. record keeping
4. radiography
5. legislation in general dental practice
6. staff training and personal training
7. risk management.

Referral letters

Referral letters also form part of the records and are important in establishing why a referral was made. Their primary purpose is to assist the recipient in making administrative decisions on accepting the referral, prioritising the referral, contacting the patient and making a suitable appointment. Studies have shown a distinct lack of crucial information, such as relevant medical histories[18] and relevant dental history.[19] In this last study, a proforma was produced which improved the quality of the referrals.

The Department of Health has issued guidance (www.doh.gov/patientsletters/issues.htm) about copying referral letters to patients, based on a government commitment in the NHS Plan in 1997 that patients should be able to receive copies of clinicians' letters about them as of right. It is considered good practice to copy patients into correspondence, as it keeps them informed. There are some provisos relating to when this is not advisable and these include:

- where the patient does not want a copy
- where the dentist feels that it may cause harm to the patient or for other reasons

- where the letter includes information about a third party who has not given consent
- where special safeguards for confidentiality may be needed.

Radiographs

Radiographs are very much part of clinical records and should be retained for the same length of time as other clinical records. Storage of these records presents two problems. Firstly, wet-film-based radiographs, if not processed properly, will rapidly discolour, and there is no information on the likely lifespan of current emulsions.[20] Secondly, while an increasing number of practitioners are mounting intra-oral radiographs, many continue to be filed, or misfiled, in envelopes from which radiographs are readily lost. Digital radiographs (attached as a file to the patient's computer records) will obviate these problems.

Radiographs should only be taken when clinically necessary, and a note of how many and the type should be recorded in the notes. It is prudent to take radiographs of any tooth that is planned for surgical extraction, root filling or extensive treatment such as crowns. Failure to take radiographs when indicated, taking poor radiographs and/or failing to check them is a common basis for findings of clinical negligence. What is also mandatory is a contemporaneous report on the radiographs.

Radiography reports

It is essential that all radiographs are reported on with dates, within the body of the clinical notes. A simple 'Checked' by the side of the record of the radiograph being taken is sufficient if nothing abnormal is detected. There is no expectation that pathology-free radiographs should be reported on in detail.

Where there is pathology, such as caries, bone loss, lesions or other factors of significance (e.g. overhanging restorations, subgingival calculus or suboptimal dental treatment), it is important these are noted. If these aspects of the radiograph are discussed with the patient, it is also important this is noted in the records.

Quality assurance of radiographs

Radiographs are an integral part of the provision of dental care, and form part of the records. The legal responsibilities for using X-ray equipment are guided by the Ionising Radiation Regulations 1999 (IRR99), which relate principally to the protection of workers and the public, and the Ionising Radiation (Medical Exposure) Regulations 2000 (IR[ME]R 2000).

The essential procedures within a quality assurance programme in general dental practice will relate to:

- image quality
- patient dose and X-ray equipment
- dark room, films and processing
- training
- audit.

Registered dentists (for the purposes of this legislation) are 'IRMER practitioners' and have to receive appropriate training, which will be covered by a UK dental degree or equivalent. Dental radiology also has to be a part of a dentist's continuing professional development (CPD). Guidance states that, whilst this CPD can be a mixture of both verifiable and general CPD within a 5-yearly cycle of 250 hours, an average practitioner would be expected to devote at least 5% of the hours to radiology and radiation protection.

A subjective quality rating of radiographs which could be a useful basis for an audit in radiography is included in Appendix 3.

How long should we keep records?

Paper records can cause enormous storage problems, and over a period of time a practice will accumulate a considerable amount. Add to this radiographs such as lateral cephalometric views and orthodontic study models, and it is not difficult to see why the limited space of a practice compounds the situation. Box 2.3 summarises the statutory requirements relevant to time limits on record keeping.

The Limitation Act provides a legal construct which controls the time a claimant has to bring an action in court after the incident complained of. The Limitation Act states that the primary limitation period in respect of personal injury is 3 years from the date on which the cause of action accrued or the date of knowledge (if later) of the injured person.

Section 14 of the 1980 Act provides that the date of knowledge, which starts the primary limitation

---

Box 2.3 Statutory acts relevant to time limits on record keeping

NATIONAL HEALTH SERVICE (GENERAL DENTAL SERVICES) REGULATIONS 1992 (AS AMENDED)
Para 25(2)
'The records, radiographs, photographs and study models (orthodontic) shall be retained for a period of 2 years after completion of any course of care and treatment under a continuing care arrangement or a capitation arrangement or treatment on referral or occasional treatment to which they relate.'

Limitation Acts
- Personal Injury: 3 years (from incident or the date of knowledge that something had gone wrong) to issue proceedings plus 4 months in which to serve proceedings
- Breach of Contract: 6 years from the date of commencement of the contract plus 4 months in which to serve proceedings
- Inland Revenue: 7 years
- NB In the case of minors, the time limits do not commence until the age of 18

Consumer Protection Act 1987
Product liability: 10 years

---

period running, is the date upon which a person first knew that he had a significant injury which was attributable, in whole or in part, to the act or omission alleged to constitute the negligence.[21]

For example, a patient may attend a new dentist, to be advised that a root canal instrument had fractured inside a canal necessitating the extraction or specialist re-treatment of the tooth. If the patient was not informed at the time of the instrument fracture, the date of knowledge will be when they are told by the new dentist of the retained instrument. This date of knowledge may be many years after the original incident occurred, but the patient can still bring a claim against their former dentist. Therefore, it could be important in defending the action that clinical records from the time of the incident are available.

Under the Consumer Protection Act 1987 there is strict liability for defective products upon producers (including manufacturers) and suppliers where the product causes physical injury (including death) or property damage. In the case of laboratory-produced items, for the purposes of this Act, the producer will be the laboratory and the supplier (under section 46) will be the dentist. The ten years limit is the maximum time within which a claim can be made, beginning with the date when the product was first put into circulation. From section 2 of the Act, the principal liability is that of the 'producer'. While a supplier may also be liable, liability can be avoided by identifying the supplier or the producer to the claimant.[22]

The Data Protection Act 1998 lays down the following guidelines for the minimum retention of records.[23]

1. Records relating to children and young people (including paediatric, vaccination and community child health records): until the patient's 25th birthday; or 26th birthday if an entry was made when the young person was 17; or 10 years after the death of a patient if sooner.
2. Records relating to those serving in HM Armed Forces: not to be destroyed.
3. Records relating to those serving a prison sentence: not to be destroyed.
4. All other personal health records: 10 years after the conclusion of treatment, the patient's death or after the patient has permanently left the country.
5. Patient records used in connection with clinical trials should be kept for at least 15 years.

Disposal of records

There is a conflicting demand between the destruction of records, which is of course permanent, and the continuing storage of records which is expensive and sometimes impractical for reasons of space. If you are destroying information, it is important that confidentiality is maintained. Specialist security firms are available to do this data disposal. However, it is important to ensure they sign a confidentiality agreement, and a written certificate is provided as proof of destruction. Paper records should be incinerated or shredded. Disk, tapes and CD-ROMs should be overwritten with random data (software is available for this purpose) or destroyed. The hard disks of computers will not have data permanently destroyed by either deleting files or reformatting the drive. Again, software can be purchased that will overwrite the drive with random data. Alternatively, the disk can be destroyed. The practice should have a written policy on the destruction of records.[24]

Unwelcome publicity is likely to follow the discovery of records on computer discs. A national newspaper report (*The Daily Telegraph* 2004) under the headline 'Medical files found in boot sale computer' highlighted the discovery of psychiatric reports of hundreds of local Essex patients written by a consultant on a hard drive sold for £4 in a car boot sale.

WHO HAS ACCESS TO CLINICAL RECORDS?

Patient access

The relevant law, as it relates to England and Wales, on controlling access to dental records is to be found in The Access to Health Records Act 1990 and The Data Protection Act 1998.

The Access to Health Records Act 1990

This Act created (for the first time) a right for patients to see their medical records. This has largely been superseded by the Data Protection Act, since now the only categories of applicant entitled to access records under this 1990 Act are the personal representatives of a patient who has died or any person who may have a claim arising out of the patient's death. Therefore, the instances when this Act is relevant in general dental practice will be few.

The Data Protection Act 1998

The Data Protection Act, which became effective from 1st March 2000, is a complex and, some say, Byzantine piece of legislation intended to protect people's privacy by preventing unauthorised or inappropriate use of their personal details. It is very wide-ranging, covering all individuals and organisations holding data about identifiable people, including healthcare records. For the purposes of the Act, a health record is any record that consists of information relating to the physical or mental health or condition of an individual, and has been made by or on behalf of a health professional in connection with the care of that individual.

In terms of access, a patient can have access to all dental records held about them, be those records on a computer or manually kept. This will include any correspondence, laboratory instructions sheets, photographs, intra-oral images and radiographs.

They should be provided promptly, within 21 days of the request being made. If it appears that providing the records may take longer than 40 days, the applicant should be informed and an explanation of the delay provided.

Access can only be refused where providing such would disclose information about someone else who has not given consent, or where disclosure would be likely to cause serious harm to the mental or physical health of the applicant or any other person. In the case of dental records this is unlikely.

Responsibility for dealing with an access to health record request lies with the 'data controller', which under the Act could be a dentist or the practice manager. The data controller is not obliged to supply any information under section 7(1) unless he has received a request in writing and except in prescribed cases, such fee (not exceeding the prescribed maximum) as he may require (see below for fees).

Children and young adults

As a general rule, a person with parental responsibility will have the right to apply for access to a child's health record. The law in England and Wales regards young people aged 16 or 17 to be adults for the purposes of consent to treatment and right to confidentiality. Therefore, if a 16-year-old wishes a dental practitioner to keep treatment confidential, that wish should be respected and access to health records could be denied to parents.

Third party access to records

Other than patients or their representatives, there are a number of other agencies that may request or have legal access to patients' records. These include insurance companies who may be paying for treatment, the police, the Inland Revenue when investigating the tax affairs of a practitioner, or the health authority or regulatory body. This will be dealt with more fully in Chapter 4 (Confidentiality).

Cost of access

The Data Protection Act 1998 clarifies the costs to access records from the holder.

- A maximum fee of £10 for granting access to health records which are automatically processed or are recorded with the intention that they are so processed.

- A maximum fee of £50 for granting access to manual records, or a mixture of manual and automated records.

This maximum charge includes both the cost of copying and administration. There is no statutory provision to allow charging for copying or postage, or to allow an individual who has not paid to inspect their own records in the event that they do not wish to obtain copies.

There is no charge allowable under the Data Protection Act where the request is restricted solely to data which forms part of a health record, and that record has been at least partially created within the 40 days preceding the request and no permanent copy of the information is to be provided. This would allow the patient to view the records at the practice without taking a copy of them.

The Data Protection Act does not entitle the patient requesting the records to have copies of the record if 'the supply of such a copy is not possible or would involve disproportionate effort'. However, this is unlikely in the case of radiographs, study models or photographs as these can be copied reasonably easily by the local hospital or other companies. If the patient is not willing to pay, there is no obligation on the practice to incur the costs themselves.

Radiographs and traces are included as part of the records, and copying them should only entail a maximum fee of £50, which will also include the charge for copying the manual records. This was confirmed in *Hubble* v. *Peterborough Hospital NHS Trust* (2001), unreported before Recorder Christopher Butler.

Refusal of access

Situations in which access to clinical records will be refused should be rare in a general dental practice situation, but these include:

- Where you believe that access to the record would disclose information likely to cause serious harm to the physical or mental health of the patients or of any other individual, which may include a health professional (e.g. terminal illness, AIDS, etc.).
- When you believe that access to the record would disclose confidential information related to or provided by an individual other than the

patient, who could be identified from that information.

- When the patient is a child (under 16) and you believe that they are capable of understanding the nature of an application made (e.g. by a parent).
- When the patient is dead and had previously requested that certain information was not to be disclosed (e.g. to the applicant).
- Where the data was obtained as a result of any examination or investigation to which the data subject consented on the basis that the information would not be disclosed.

If a practice refuses access unreasonably under the Data Protection Act, an application to the county court to order disclosure can be made by the patient's solicitors, or a complaint can be made to the Information Commissioner.

Freedom of Information Act 2000

NHS dentists are included in the scope of 'public authorities' as defined in the Act and as such have to comply with the Act from November 2003. The Freedom of Information Act is intended to promote greater openness and accountability across the public sector and every NHS practice has to adopt and maintain a 'publication scheme' which has been approved by the Information Commissioner (www.informationcommisioner.gov.uk).

In relation to clinical records, any official caught shredding or defacing e-mails or records they know to be requested by a member of the public wanting to view their private files will commit a crime. Under this legislation, a healthcare worker could face fines of up to £5000 for 'altering, erasing or defacing' documents requested under the Data Protection Act. This is a recognition that, once made, the records in a sense 'belong' to the patients.

The Data Protection Act provides patients and employees with the right of access to personal information held about them. The right applies to all information held in computerised form and non-computerised information held in filing systems. This is known as the subject access right. Application for access by third parties is made under the Freedom of Information Act but this cannot override the confidentiality of personal health information. These would constitute

exemptions, although the majority will be related to the public interest test.

Exemptions relevant to dentists are:

- investigations and proceedings conducted by public authorities
- personal information
- commercial interests
- information provided in confidence.

Who owns the clinical records?

In the case of NHS records, true ownership of the notes probably lies in the ownership of the paper upon which they are written. In the case of general dental practitioner notes, the FP25 records are the property of the NHS and the owner would be the relevant primary care trust/health board. In the case of private record cards, the ownership would lie with the purchaser of those blank record cards—the practice owner, be it an individual or corporate.

This question arises often in disputes between clinicians who may leave a practice and then continue to treat a patient somewhere else. In reality, the fact of ownership does not provide an excuse from refraining from providing disclosure under the Access to Health Records Act 1990 or the Data Protection Act 1998, should the patient themselves request it.

The ownership of radiographs is slightly more problematic in that the practice owner purchases the film and owns the chemicals or equipment used in processing that film. A private patient may argue to be the rightful owner, as they have in fact paid for it as an individual item of treatment. The contrary view is that the patient pays for the opinion and diagnosis, not the radiograph itself, and therefore ownership rights do not accrue to the patient.

The radiographs, in any case, form part of the dental records and should not be separated from them.

ELECTRONIC DENTAL RECORDS

The electronic dental record has been given impetus by the government's desire to allow medical patients in the NHS to be treated seamlessly in either primary care or secondary care and geographically anywhere in the UK. The obvious benefit is that healthcare professionals in a multidisciplinary environment will have instant access to a patient's previous or current records and diagnostic information. The technology is there and affordable, and patients are coming to expect it.

In general practice, this electronic patient record (EPR) would have the benefit of a referral being made to a specialist for hospital, and information can be shared electronically regardless of geography. A patient's progress can be tracked, and consultations and diagnosis can be made with the help of digital images and radiographs.

The intention is to create a 'spine record' for every patient, holding essential information anyone making health decisions about that patient needs to know. It will also allow patients to know what information is being shared about them and who is seeing it. Eventually, patients will be able to view their records in their own homes via a well-protected internet link.[25]

Patients are now able to access their own records by scanning their thumbprints into a reader, without the need for passwords or pin numbers. This Patient Access Electronic Record System (PAERS) allows access to a patient's records as well as the appointment book, and is being piloted in general medical practices in London.

There are some serious considerations about confidentiality and the availability of patient-sensitive data from sites quite remote from where they were collected if the EPRs are populated with the patient NHS number. This will allow authorised users to access information about the patient's medical and dental treatment and condition anywhere there is access to the NHS net across the UK.[26]

FURTHER READING

Faculty of General Dental Practitioners (UK). Clinical Examination and Record Keeping, Good Practice Guidelines. London: Faculty of General Dental Practitioners (UK); 2001.

Field EA, Longman LP. Guidance for the management of natural latex allergy in dental patients and dental healthcare workers. London: Faculty of General Dental Practitioners (UK); 2004.

Howard P, Hall J. Guide to the coursework module of the MFGDP(UK) examination. London: Faculty of General Dental Practitioners (UK); 2002.

National Radiological Protection Board. Guidance notes for dental practitioners on the safe use of X-ray equipment. National Radiological Protection Board; 2001. (www.nrpb.org.uk)

Pendlebury ME, Horner K, Eaton KA, eds. Selection criteria for dental radiography. 2nd edn. London: Faculty of General Dental Practitioners; 2004.

Rattan R, Chambers R, Wakley G. Clinical governance in general dental practice. Abingdon: Radcliffe Medical Press; 2002.

REFERENCES

1 Watt R, McGlone P, Evans D et al. The facilitating factors and barriers influencing change in dental practice in a sample of English general dental practitioners. BDJ 2004; 197: 485–489.

2 Burke FJT, Wilson NHF. Measuring oral health: an historical view and details of a contemporary oral health index (OHX). Int Dent J 1995; 45:358–370.

3 Delargy S. Providing a numerical measure of oral health—can it be done and how accurate is it? Dent Update 2004; 31:457–460.

4 Clark DH. An analysis of the value of forensic odontology in ten mass disasters. Int Dent J 1994; 44:241–250.

5 Liss G, Sussman G. Latex sensitisation: occupational versus general population prevalence rates. Am J Indust Med 1999; 25:196–200.

6 Croser D. Periodic needs. Dental Practice Magazine. November 2004: 39. www.dentalpracticeuk.net

7 Standards for Dental Professionals. General Dental Council. June 2005. www.gdc-uk.org

8 Peer Review and Clinical Audit in General Dental Practice. London: Department of Health 1997.

9 Health Act 1999 Explanatory Notes. Chapter 8. HMSO: 70.

10 Marshall KF. Evaluating quality through records and radiographs—a rationale for general dental practice. Br Dent J 1995; 179:234–235.

11 Smith JM, Farrington CA. It ain't what you say—legibility and clarity of treatment records. Dent Update 2000; 27:384–386.

12 Crawford JR, Beresford TP, Lafferty KL. The CRABEL score—a method for auditing medical records. Ann R Coll Surg Engl 2001; 83:65–68.

13 Computerised Records. Risk Management module 28. DPL Publications. www.dentalprotection.org

14 Morgan RG. Quality evaluation of clinical records of a group of general dental practitioners entering a quality assurance programme. Br Dent J 2001; 191:436–441.

15 Rasmusson L, Rene N, Dahlbom U and Borrman H. Quality evaluation of patient records in Swedish dental care. Swed Dent J 1994; 18:233–241.

16 Pessian F, Beckett HA. Record keeping by undergraduate dental students: a clinical audit. Br Dent J 2004; 197:703–705.

17 Chasteen J, Cameron C, Phillips S. An audit system for assessing dental record keeping. J Dent Ed 1996; 60(129): 78-987.

18 Chambers I, Scully C. Medical information from referral letters. Oral Surg Oral Med Oral Path 1987; 64(6):674–676.

19 Djemal S, Chia M, Ubaye–Narayange T. Quality improvement of referrals to a department of restorative dentistry following the use of a referral pro forma by referring dentist. Br Dent J 2004; 197(2):85–88.

20 Hirschman PN. Transfer of radiographs. Br Dent J 1999; 187(9):463-464.

21 Green M, McConnochie K. Clinical negligence and complaints: a clinician's guide. London: Royal Society of Medicine; 2002.

22 Kennedy I, Grubb A. Medical Law. 3rd edn. London: Butterworths; 2000.

23 NHS Executive. HSC 1998/217: Preservation, retention and destruction of GP general medical services records relating to patients. NHS Executive; 2001.

24 Medical Protection Society. Keeping medical records. Medical Protection Society; 2002.

25 Consumers Association/NHS National Programme for Information Technology. The Public View on Electronic Health Records. Health Which? And NHS National Programme for Information Technology; Oct 2003.

26 Department of Health, RCGP, BMA. Good practice guidelines for GP electronic patient records (Version 3). Department of Health; 2003.

Consent—getting to yes

3

'*Every person being of adult years and sound mind has a right to determine what shall be done with his own body.*'

J. Cardozo in Schloendorff v. Society of New York Hospital (1914)

This is the starting point for consent, establishing the doctrine of autonomy (literally self rule) in which a patient is entitled to come to any decision about their treatment or refusal of treatment, freely and independently. Whilst the dentist's role is to help a patient come to a decision by providing information and choices, ultimately the decision should be the patient's alone.

Recognising an individual's right of autonomy makes self-creation possible. It allows each of us to be responsible for shaping our lives according to our own coherent (or incoherent, but in any case, distinctive) personality. It allows us to lead our lives rather than be led along them, so that each of us can be, to the extent a scheme of rights can make this possible, what we have made of ourselves.[1]

In extremis, 'Even when his or her life depends on receiving medical treatment, an adult of sound mind is entitled to refuse it' (*St Georges Healthcare NHS Trust* v. *S*).[2] And in a similar vein: 'An adult patient has an absolute right to refuse to consent to medical treatment for any reason, rational or irrational, or for no reason at all, even where that decision may lead to his death'(Re MB).[3]

Whilst such a situation is unlikely to be faced by a dentist in general practice the principle remains paramount. A patient can refuse treatment offered, even if it is in the patient's best interests. The Human Rights Act 1998 also creates obligations for clinicians, and Article 8 (the right to respect for privacy, family life and correspondence) and Article 10 (the right to freedom of expression including the right to receive and impart information) are likely to be engaged in the issue of consent.

It is a 'fundamental principle, now long established, that every person's body is inviolate' (Lord Goff in Re F *[Mental patient sterilisation]*).[4] A patient's freedom to consent and make a decision about his or her own body is constrained by the choices given by the dentist in clinical practice, and the patient cannot demand whatever treatment they wish. Furthermore, a patient cannot compel a dentist to provide treatment that is judged by that clinician not to be in the patient's best interests.

BATTERY

Failure to obtain consent before touching someone constitutes battery, for which damages may be awarded in civil law and which, in extreme cases, constitutes the criminal offence of assault. This was summarised in a House of Lords decision: 'Prima facie, therefore, in the absence of consent all, or almost all, medical treatment and all surgical treatment of an adult is unlawful, however beneficial such treatment might be. This is incontestable' (Lord Donaldson in Re F).[5]

In reality, the courts are very reluctant to frame actions against healthcare professionals in terms of trespass and battery, as battery is an intentional action whereas most claims for injury in a clinical context involve allegations of negligence or carelessness. Dentists are most often acting in good faith. The threshold to avoid a claim for battery is quite low, in that all that is required is to provide information in broad terms as opposed to the detail which would be required to obtain consent as part of a dentist's duty of care.

This approach was firmly established by Bristow in *Chatterton* v. *Gerson*[6]: 'In my judgement once the patient is informed in broad terms of the nature of the procedure which is intended, and gives her consent, that consent is real, and the cause of action on which to base a claim for failure to go into risks and implications is negligence, not trespass'.

For example, where a dentist has recommended the removal of a tooth for an abscess, in order for the patient consent to be valid (from the point of view of avoiding battery), the dentist would need to inform the patient that a local anaesthetic would be required, the tooth would be removed and that it would heal up. It would not be necessary to give any information about the risks, benefits or alternative treatments, although this would be essential to avoid a claim of negligence.

Nevertheless, in the only reported dental case in England, a dentist was found guilty of battery by reason of lack of consent to treatment on those teeth that required no treatment (*Appleton and Others* v. *Garrett*)[7]. In this case, it was proved that the dentist deliberately withheld information that the treatment was unnecessary because he knew that the patients would not have consented had they known the true position. The patients were awarded aggravated damages. Long and expensive courses of treatment involving fillings, root fillings and crowns were carried out, often on virgin teeth, in young patients. Thus, if information is withheld in bad faith, the consent will be vitiated by fraud.

NATURE OF CONSENT

Consent to treatment may be implied or expressed.

Implied consent

Many patients do not explicitly give express consent but their agreement may be implied by compliant actions.[8] Patients who attend your surgery for a check-up or in pain imply their consent to an examination of their mouth by sitting in the chair and opening their mouth. They have consented to nothing else, and in order to carry out any invasive procedure, such as periodontal probing, percussion or vitality tests or a radiographic examination, express consent is required.

Express consent

Express consent is given when patients confirm their agreement to a procedure or treatment in clear and explicit terms, whether orally or in writing. There is no requirement in English law that consent should be in writing, but it is considered

good practice in certain procedures, such as surgical extractions of impacted wisdom teeth or implant placements. However, written consent on its own without an explanation is insufficient, and certainly the usual catch-all clause relating to 'any additional procedures deemed necessary' will only be valid in certain circumstances.

There are three essential components to valid consent:

- **Competence:** means that the patient has sufficient ability to understand the nature of the treatment and the consequences of receiving or declining that treatment. The legal term is capacity.
- **Voluntariness:** means that the patient has fully agreed to have the treatment and there has been no coercion or undue influence to accept or decline the treatment.
- **Information and knowledge:** means that sufficient comprehensible information is disclosed to the patient regarding the nature and consequences of the proposed and alternative treatments.

All these three elements are interdependent but must be present for consent to be ethically and legally valid.

Consent is not a single event but a process, and a good working definition from the UK Department of Health is as follows:

'The voluntary continuing permission of the patient to receive particular treatments. It must be based upon the patient's adequate knowledge of the purpose, nature, likely effects and risks of that treatment including the likelihood of its success and a discussion of any alternative to it including no treatment.'[9]

The emphasis on 'continuing permission' is important. For example, consider a patient requiring molar root canal therapy. If during the procedure a difficulty is encountered, such as a curved or sclerosed canal, further consent is required if the success of the therapy may be compromised and the prevailing situation is different from when treatment commenced. This further consent procedure enables the patient to weigh up the risk of continuing (or leaving the canal unfilled) against a decision to extract the tooth.

Communication and consent must go hand in hand if the patient is to be provided with sufficient information to give continued permission for a particular treatment. Once given, a patient may withdraw consent at any time, including during the performance of a procedure.[10]

CAPACITY

Before a patient can give valid consent to dental treatment, they must be deemed in law to possess the required capacity. The approach to capacity both ethically and legally is a 'functional' one driven by the process of how the patient comes to a decision. It can also be described as a cognitive test.

The test of capacity is that the person concerned should have the ability to understand the nature and purpose of the proposed care, and there is a presumption that adults over 18 years old have a capacity to consent. Patients aged 16 and 17 years old in England and Wales, by virtue of the Family Law Reform Act 1969, are also presumed to have capacity:

> 'The consent of a minor who has attained the age of 16 years old to any surgical, medical or dental treatment which, in the absence of consent, would constitute a trespass to his person, shall be as effective as it would be if he were of full age; and where a minor has by virtue of this section given an effective consent to any treatment it shall not be necessary to obtain any consent for it from his parent or guardian…'[11]

In children below the age of 16, the capacity to consent to treatment is a matter of clinical judgement based on the degree of intelligence and understanding of the child to make the relevant decision—Gillick competence (see case history below).

Assessing capacity

Every person is presumed to have the capacity to consent to or refuse medical treatment unless and until that presumption is rebutted.[13] Because an adult who is deemed to have capacity can make any decision they wish in terms of how they should be treated no matter how bizarre or how little that decision would be in their best interest, the test for capacity is an important one. The vast majority of patients attending the average general dental practice for treatment would be deemed to have capacity, but there are important steps to test that capacity.[14]

1. *Providing the information in order to make the decision*

    Exactly what information should be provided will be considered later, but here it is important that the patient:

    - recognises that a decision has to be made about treatment
    - understands in broad terms the nature of the treatment

The Gillick case[12]

Mrs Gillick had five daughters, all under the age of 16. A government circular from the Department of Health and Social Security was sent to doctors indicating that in the exceptional case of a girl under 16 attending a family planning clinic for contraceptive advice and treatment, providing such advice and treatment would not be unlawful as long as the doctor was acting in good faith to protect the girl from the harmful effects of sexual intercourse. The circular also said it was permissible to prescribe the contraceptive pill without the consent of the girl's parents under appropriate circumstances. Mrs Gillick sought an assurance from the health authority that her own daughters would not be given any contraceptive advice or treatment without her prior knowledge.

The health authority declined to give that assurance and the case went from the High Court to the Court of Appeal (who reversed the decision) and then subsequently on to the House of Lords—the final arbiter in the matter. The judges, including the late Lord Scarman, made it clear that a child under the age of 16 who had sufficient understanding to know what was being proposed was more than capable of consenting to a wide range of treatment irrespective of the parents' wishes.

As Lord Scarman declared: 'It will be a question of fact whether a child seeking advice has sufficient understanding of what is involved to give consent valid in law. Until the child achieves the capacity to consent, the parental right to make the decision continues save only in exceptional circumstances. Emergency, parental neglect, abandonment of the child or inability to find the parent are examples of exceptional situations justifying the doctor proceeding to treat the patient without parental knowledge and consent'.

- understands the principal benefits and risks of that treatment
- understands the consequences of not having the proposed treatment.

2. *Assessing the patient's cognitive ability*

Once the patient has been given the information, the next step in assessing the capacity to give consent is to ensure:

- they can understand and retain the information
- they believe it
- they are able to weigh that information and balance the risk against the advantages and make a decision.

The requirements for patient understanding vary considerably with the complexity of the decision at hand. Some decisions in clinical dentistry may require a low level of competence, such as whether or not to carry out a filling when there is a hole in a tooth visible clinically and obvious to the patient. Other decisions will demand a much higher level of understanding or 'processing' of the information and, therefore, may be more difficult for a younger patient or mentally disabled adult (see case history below).

VOLUNTARINESS

The second element of consent is that it should be voluntary and freely given without coercion. A consent obtained by misrepresentation or fraud is legally viewed as no consent at all, and from an ethical point of view there can be no moral authorisation for treatment since it violates the patient's dignity and right to self determination.

This coercion may be subtle, ranging from issues of quality, price and value, and may be influenced by the practice environment, the dentist's personality or other team members. Of course, the coercion may be exercised with benevolent intentions where the practitioner and patient differ in their assessments of how the patient's welfare is best served,[16] and in this case it would be difficult to argue that consent has been vitiated.

The test case in English law in which the issue of a patient's consent was said to be unduly influenced by someone else was Re T (see case history below).

Whilst this case deals with the refusal of consent, more commonly in practice the situation arises when a patient has apparently agreed but may claim that the consent was not freely given. Thus, 'undue influence' on the patients who may agree to a course of treatment may vitiate any consent that was given.

> '*It is wholly acceptable that the patient should have been persuaded by others of the merits of a decision and have decided accordingly. It matters not how strong the persuasion was, so long as it did not overbear the independence of the patient's decision.*'

Lord Donaldson MR *(Re T)*

Legal case for test of adult capacity: *Re C*[15]

C, a man of Jamaican origin, was sentenced at the Old Bailey to 7 years imprisonment in 1962, following the stabbing of his ex-partner. Whilst serving the sentence, he was diagnosed as suffering from chronic paranoid schizophrenia and was transferred to Broadmoor. There he stayed and mellowed with age. In 1993, C (now aged 68) presented with an ulcerated foot which was diagnosed to be gangrenous and a consultant vascular surgeon at nearby Heatherwood Hospital advised amputation below the right knee, without which C only had a 15% chance of living. C refused to give his consent to the amputation, preferring to die if necessary with both legs rather than one. He consented to conservative treatment under general anaesthetic, but there still remained a risk of death. The hospital applied to the court to have his leg amputated in the eventuality it was required without the patient's consent, on the basis that he lacked the capacity to understand the implications. Meanwhile, C trusted in his own decision, believing he was right, that God was on his side and that (believing in his delusional state) his international career in medicine in which he never lost a patient would stand him in good stead.

In his judgement, the judge granted the injunction to C, preventing the hospital from now or in the future amputating his leg without his consent. The judge did so accepting that C had capacity on the three-stage test described:

- comprehend and retain the relevant information
- believe it
- weigh it in the balance so as to arrive at a choice.

Re T (adult refusal of treatment)[17]

In 1992, Miss T, an adult and then 34-weeks pregnant, was involved in a road traffic accident. She was admitted to hospital some days later with chest pains, diagnosed as pleurisy or pneumonia. Although brought up by her mother, a fervent Jehovah's witness, Miss T was not a member of that faith and her paternal family, with whom she was living, was opposed to the sect.

The following day, after a visit from her mother and whilst in considerable pain, coughing sputum and in the early stages of labour, she said she did not want a blood transfusion if it became necessary. She signed a form to this effect but it was not explained to her that it might be necessary to give a blood transfusion to prevent injury to her health or even to save her life. The baby was delivered by caesarean section but was stillborn, and that night Miss T's condition deteriorated, following an abscess in her lungs. Her condition in intensive care was critical and a transfusion was given.

The Court of Appeal judges agreed that it was lawful to give the blood transfusion because Miss T was unduly influenced by her mother and would not have refused the transfusion had her mother not been there.

KNOWLEDGE

The essential component of the knowledge element is how much information a patient needs to know about a particular dental procedure in order for the consent to be valid and, therefore, defensible in any negligence action brought by the patient.

The most important case that demonstrates how English law deals with this aspect of consent is the Sidaway case (see below).

This is completely different from the United States of America where the law requires that the patient is given all the relevant information, leading to sometimes bizarre consent forms in which every risk known is disclosed.

However, it is clear even in English law that the patient should be given sufficient information in order to make an informed choice.

So what information should be given to a patient contemplating treatment?

- The patient must be informed of any serious risk, even if of low frequency
- The patient should be warned about transient and less serious risks that occur more commonly.

The duty to disclose is, to some extent, dependent upon the risk:benefit ratio of treatment. So in aesthetic procedures, failure to disclose even remote risks may be difficult to justify. Ultimately, however, the Bolam test (see p. 59) still applies, where a dentist will not be found negligent if he has acted in accordance with the practice accepted as proper by a responsible body of dentists. In other words, if it is not generally appropriate to warn about something, a dentist cannot be found guilty of negligence if he fails to warn. This has been slightly modified by the Bolitho case[19] in which it was said that the 'responsible body' relied upon by any defendant must demonstrate that an opinion should have a *logical* basis.

For example the US, Australia, South Africa and Ireland apply the *objective standard* and the *subjective standard*, both of which are different from the UK standard which is the *professional test* of whether a warning should be given. In the objective standard, the question is what a reasonable or 'prudent' patient would expect to be told about a procedure in order to make a decision. The subjective standard is more patient-focused

Sidaway[18]

Mrs Sidaway suffered from pain in her neck, right shoulder and arms, and underwent an operation designed to relieve her symptoms. Prior to the operation, the surgeon explained to her that there was a 1–2% chance of damage to the spinal column and the nerve roots where they emerged from the spinal column. However, the risk of damage to the spinal cord itself was not mentioned prior to surgery. Unfortunately, Mrs Sidaway's spinal column was damaged in procedure, leaving her severely disabled after the operation. Her claim for negligence was based on her assertion that the surgeon had failed to disclose or explain all the risks inherent in the operation. When eventually the case came before the House of Lords, Mrs. Sidaway was unable to prove her case, but the Court availed themselves of the opportunity to explain a doctor's duty under the circumstances. They rejected the concept of 'informed consent', saying this was totally impractical, and held it was a matter of clinical judgement whether a risk should be disclosed or not to the patient.

again, and here it is a question of what would be important to a particular patient with regard to the risks of the treatment being proposed at that particular time.

Cases since Sidaway are suggesting that the English courts will increasingly be expecting clinicians to provide information required by the 'prudent' patient. In *Pearce* v. *United Bristol Healthcare Trust*, Lord Woolf MR concluded that 'if there is a significant risk which would affect the judgement of a reasonable patient, then in the normal course it is the responsibility of a doctor to inform the patient of that significant risk, if the information is needed so that the patient can determine for himself or herself as to what course he or she should adopt'.[20] In this case, the claimant, who was expecting her sixth child, was overdue by two weeks and requested her consultant to have an induced labour or caesarean section. The consultant advised her to let nature take its course, but the child died in utero a week later and was stillborn.

The question was whether the consultant should have advised Mrs Pearce about the risk of stillbirth if she waited, and whether that information would have altered her decision to have a natural birth. In this case, the risk of stillbirth was something like 0.1–0.2% and therefore could by no means be considered a significant risk. Therefore, the Court of Appeal agreed that since the risk was not significant there was no duty to disclose it.

What level of risk?

This raises the question then of what is the threshold above which a risk should be disclosed to a patient in order for them to make a decision. In the Sidaway case, it was suggested by one of the lawlords that a 10% risk of a side-effect is a 'significant risk' and that it should be disclosed to the patient as part of the consent procedure. That is the starting point, but whether a risk is significant or not cannot be determined simply in terms of percentages. It must be considered in relation to what a 'reasonable patient' would consider relevant to their decision.

In *Chester* v. *Afshar*,[21] the neurosurgeon Mr Afshar was found negligent for failing to warn his patient Miss Chester of a small but unavoidable risk of 1-2% of the surgery leading to the seriously adverse result of cauda equina syndrome. Both sides agreed there was no negligence in the actual manner in which the surgery was carried out. This case has proved to be a significant change in the doctrine of informed consent in English law.

The patient, Miss Chester, could not state that, had she been given a proper warning as to the risks of cauda equina, she would never have had the operation. All she could have said was that she would have discussed matters with others and explored alternative options. In other words, the operation would not have proceeded on *that* Monday, but she might have agreed to have it performed at a later date, perhaps even by Mr Afshar himself. The risk on any such future occasion would have been the same, i.e. 1-2 %.

This decision has serious implications for clinicians. Failure to take adequate consent—and recording it—now overrides any argument that such failure did not cause the adverse outcome, provided that the warning ought to have been given and the condition or consequence which ought to have been mentioned actually develops.[22] It will no longer be sufficient to record 'warned of risks' or the equivalent, which may leave dentists vulnerable. As highlighted in the above case, a detailed account of the specific risks about which a patient is warned ought to replace common shorthand notes.

Informed consent requires the imparting of information that the patient would expect to know before agreeing to undergo a procedure. Permanent impairment of everyday activities, such as speaking, would certainly fall into this category. Leaflets specific to certain procedures are a useful way of outlining major and significant risks, and it must be documented in the notes that the relevant information was given and discussed in this form. It is important also to recognise that the complications of a procedure that might have a specific effect on a patient's lifestyle (e.g. restrict the patient's ability to work) may also have a significant effect on willingness to undergo a particular procedure.[23]

Information about the level of risk in any particular aspect of clinical dentistry comes from peer-reviewed journals. These may or may not be related to a particular type of practice, and therefore, to overcome this, a dentist ought to consider carrying out their own clinical audit on various aspects of dental care.

Referral for general anaesthesia

In November 1998, the GDC introduced guidelines for dental practitioners when referring patients for general anaesthesia (GA). The referring practitioner has to consider other means of pain and anxiety control, and behavioural management. If these are not viable or successful, only then should GA be considered an option. The referring practitioner also has the responsibility of discussing with the patient, parent or guardian the risks involved with GA, and alternative methods of pain and anxiety control. The letter of referral should also contain a clear justification for providing GA.

Whilst this is good practice, the legal doctrine of consent requires informed consent at the time of the procedure. This becomes the clear responsibility of the team carrying out the procedure, and in a referral to secondary care or a specialist service, such treatment may be undertaken a long period after the initial decision to refer. The referral by the dentist in general practice is made on the basis that the patient understands in broad terms the purpose, nature, likely effects, risks and alternatives, but with the proviso that a full assessment will be made by the anaesthetist whose responsibility it ultimately is to ensure that appropriate consent has been obtained.

Nevertheless, research in this area found that 66% of patients who were referred for GA felt they were not informed of any of the risks of GA by their referring dentist, and 63% of letters of referral contained no reason or justification for the referral.[24] Another study in relation to GA showed that 40% of the written consent obtained from the parents were not valid. The time interval between the consent process and the actual treatment did not have any significant effect on the subjects' understanding of the consent, but the results implied that with time the subjects' knowledge actually improved.[25]

Understanding the information

Delivering the information to the patient is one thing; whether or not they understand it is another matter altogether. To avoid a charge of battery the 'law in effect places on a clinician a strict duty to explain to his patient, in language which the patient can understand, the essential nature and purpose of the treatment he is to undergo'. To avoid negligence liability, the dentist must have taken 'sufficient care to convey to the patient and *assure* that the patient *understood* the gravity, nature and extent of risks specifically attendant on the procedure'(*Reibl* v. *Hughes*).[26] Whilst this is a Canadian case, a similar line was followed in the Court of Appeal's decision in *Lybert* v. *Warrington*,[27] where a warning to avoid sex following a sterilisation procedure was given but the doctor should have taken reasonable steps to ensure the couple understood the risks in their specific case.

Clinical examples in dentistry

Aesthetic dentistry is by and large elective treatment, and therefore any attendant risks must be explained to the patient. Veneers, for example, may require large amounts of tooth reduction to be aesthetic, and the patient must be advised that they would feel bulky in the initial stages. Crown and bridgework carries a risk of the loss of vitality, and this is particularly true when misaligned teeth are being prepared to accept crowns. Where there is a high risk, the patient must be informed to allow them to make a reasoned decision.

Patients often ask about the likelihood of success in cosmetic treatment, or require some guarantees. The possibility of a contractual warranty is important since no such duty arises in negligence: the only obligation of the dentist is to act reasonably.[28] In any private care, a contractual relationship will exist between the dentist and the patient, and the terms of that contract will be for the two parties to agree. It would be unusual to guarantee a particular outcome, although certain aspects, such as the laboratory-constructed items, may carry a free replacement warranty in the event of failure within a given time period.

Nothing is for life, and patients may have unreal expectations about how long restorative work will last. It is incumbent on the dentist to provide sufficient information to allow patients to make up their minds before proceeding with any particular treatment.

Records

An essential part of the consent process is giving patients options to enable them to make a decision. When giving that information, it needs to be in language that is easy to understand and free of jargon. Leaflets are very useful to aid in this process of delivering information. Pictures, models and intra-oral images all help build up the information bank required by the patient in the consent process.

Once a decision has been made it is important to properly record this. Where more complex treatment is to be provided (especially with a higher risk of failure or when a patient is electing for treatment not recommended by the dentist), a letter with a written quote is essential.

Private versus NHS work

As part of the consent process, patients need to be given information about the quality of the treatment, if specifically requested. This will often arise in any discussion with a patient about the differences between NHS crowns or dentures and private ones. In some cases, there is no equivalent choice available on the NHS, as occurs with porcelain bonded to metal crowns on molars. However, for other options where there is a difference in materials, quality of fit and aesthetics, the patient has a right to know the differences in an objective summary of the nature of NHS crowns, bridges and dentures. This should be an essential part of the process in which information is imparted to the patient during a consultation.

Part of NHS documentation is an FP17DC form, which is a written treatment plan outlining costs. This form is useful when both NHS and private treatment are being offered to the patient, but it is not a consent form. In a study, 79% of patients mistakenly thought that signing an FP17 claim form was a consent to treatment, and it appears from other studies that two-thirds of general practitioners also think this is the case.[29] This other form (FP17) has the function of confirming the patient's agreement to pay the NHS charge, verifies that the treatment indicated is complete, and allows information to be disclosed by other agencies for counter-fraud purposes. However, it is not a consent form, and neither are any of the PDS (Personal Dental Services) forms.

In respect of costs, the GDC makes it clear that a patient should know:

- the nature of the contract and in particular whether the patient is being accepted for treatment under the NHS or privately
- the charge for an initial consultation and the probable cost of subsequent treatment

See Appendix 5 for the GDC guidance on consent.

WHEN THINGS GO WRONG

Treatment does not always go to plan. This may range simply from a contact point in a multi-surface restoration not being tight, to implants failing to osseo-integrate. It is important the patient is fully informed no matter how embarrassing such a disclosure is likely to be. The patient has a legal right to know that a particular unexpected outcome has occurred, even if it was avoidable and may potentially undermine the patient's confidence in you.

Separating instrument in canals is a well-recognised complication of root canal therapy. Fortunately, it does not occur often, which means there is no obligation to advise the patient of a risk of it occurring unless they specifically ask or the canal anatomy suggests it may be a risk factor in that particular endodontic treatment. If an instrument does separate in the canal, part of the consent process is to inform the patient and advise them of the options available, which will include a referral to a specialist. It is equally important to record this conversation on the clinical notes, confirming what option the patient took at the time. All too often this vital piece of the jigsaw is missing, and several years later when a costly referral to a specialist is finally made, possibly by another dentist, the patient refuses adamantly to accept they had declined an earlier referral.

Consent is about treating patients with courtesy and respect, recognising their dignity and rights as individuals. It is a process rather than a one-off event, and as the GDC describes: 'it should be part of an ongoing dialogue between you and the patient'.

In summary, for consent to be informed, the following information should be provided:

- what treatment is proposed and what it involves in broad terms
- why the treatment is necessary and the consequences of no treatment
- what the alternative options for treatment are and the risks associated with them
- what, if any, adverse anticipated risks there are
- what the costs are.

CHILDREN AND CONSENT

More often than not, children will attend a dental practice with their parents, usually as a family, and this is certainly something to be encouraged by the practice. It is important clinically, since oral health messages can be delivered to patient, parent and siblings equally effectively, but it also ensures issues of consent for investigations and treatment can be dealt with quickly and efficiently.

Children themselves want to be involved in the decision-making process, and they want this to be in the form of a discussion between the dentist, their parents and themselves. Children want adults to recognise and help promote their evolving autonomy by listening to them and acknowledging their contribution in consenting to dental care. This increases their understanding and satisfaction with their dental care.[30]

In the rare cases of child abuse, when oro-facial signs may give rise to suspicions, dental practitioners have an ethical and moral duty to investigate the matter, and consent becomes a matter of importance.

When is a child not a child? The first yardstick is statute law.

Children aged 16 and 17

A person under the age of 18 is considered a minor by law. In England and Wales (but not Scotland), The Family Law Reform Act 1969 sets out the position for 16- and 17-year-olds.

> '…the consent of a minor who has attained the age of sixteen years to any surgical, medical or dental treatment which, in the absence of consent, would constitute a trespass to his person, shall be as effective as it would be if he were of full age [i.e. aged 18 years or above]; and it shall not be necessary to obtain any consent for it from his parent or guardian'.

This means that in many respects they should be treated as adults—for example if a signature on a consent form is necessary, they can sign for themselves if they are deemed competent.[31] The test for competency/capacity is the same for adults (as described above). It is still good practice to encourage competent children to involve their families in decision-making processes, and where treatment incurs charges to the patient this is doubly important.

If a 16- to 17-year-old patient refuses consent for treatment that is considered to be in the patient's best interest, the Family Law Reform Act 1969 allows a person with parental responsibility to give proxy consent. In reality, it would be very difficult to physically force dental treatment on a competent 16- to 17-year-old, and since in most cases not providing dental treatment would not be life threatening, it would not be justifiable.

If a child of 16 or 17 is not competent to take a particular decision, then a person with parental responsibility (see below) can take that decision for them, although the child should still be involved as much as possible.

When children reach the age of 18, no other person can make a decision on their behalf if they are deemed to have capacity.

Children under 16

The second yardstick for deciding whether a child can give consent is measured against the Gillick case (above), which arises from common law. This allows the dentist to provide treatment in the child's best interest, in the absence of parental permission, where the child is assessed as 'Gillick competent' and has given consent for the procedure.

Case law has not shed much light on assessing Gillick competence, leaving the dentist to decide whether the child has sufficient understanding and intelligence to fully understand what is being proposed. Where interventions are minor, such as fissure sealants, it is easier to presume competence. Where, for example, choices are available, such as amalgam versus composite fillings, and parents may have concerns about certain types of restorations, it is better to discuss this with the parents.

Orthodontics is an important area where sometimes complex treatment is provided to this age group, and full discussion with a person who has parental responsibility is important. If a Gillick-competent child under 16 refuses orthodontic treatment, which they are entitled to do, even under the Children's Act 1989, it would be unwise to override that consent at the parent's insistence, since long-term patient cooperation is a significant aspect of successful orthodontic treatment.

Similarly, if a parent or someone with parental responsibility refuses treatment that a dentist believes is appropriate, a Court may be asked to decide what is in the child's best interest. This would only be when providing the treatment against the wishes of the child or parent was crucial, i.e. the child would die or suffer serious permanent injury without it. Such circumstances rarely, if ever, occur in a dental practice.

Since the assessment of Gillick competence is a developmental concept and can vary considerably, no age bands are given as guidance, although it is unlikely that the courts would consider children of 13 years or less to be Gillick competent in most situations.[32]

Parental responsibility

Who has parental responsibility is a key aspect of obtaining consent from a child. In many cases, more than one person has parental responsibility for the child (typically the natural parents), and it is important to remember that consent only has to come from one individual with parental responsibility. There is no obligation on the dentist to seek the consent of any other person with parental responsibility before providing treatment.

Issues of parental responsibility often arise either when the child is brought to the practice by a grandparent, childminder or relative, or when the parents are separating and the oral health of the child (or lack of it) is a matter of dispute. Where there is disagreement between parents about what treatment should be provided, one consenting and the other refusing, the dentist 'will be presented with a professional and ethical dilemma but not with a legal problem because if he has the consent of one authorised person, the treatment will not without more constitute a trespass or criminal assault'.[33]

The Children Act 1989 sets out who has parental responsibility and these include:

1. the child's parents if married to each other at the time of conception or birth
2. the child's mother
3. the child's father:
   a) only if he was married to the child's mother at the time of conception or birth
   b) if not so married, then he only has parental responsibility *if* he has acquired it via a court order *or* a 'parental responsibility agreement' with the mother *or* he subsequently marries the mother *or* he is named on the child's birth certificate (this new amendment comes via The Adoption and Children Act 2002)
4. the child's legally appointed guardian (appointed either by a court or by a parent with parental responsibility in the event of his or her own death)
5. a person in whose favour a court has made a residence order concerning the child
6. a local authority or other person who holds an emergency protection order in respect of the child.

Parental responsibility cannot be surrendered or transferred, but the person with parental responsibility can arrange some or all of it to be met by one or more people acting on his or her behalf. Thus, for example, parents might give authority to grandparents or a childminder to give consent under defined circumstances, such as dental treatment. Where such explicit authority has been given (and it need not be in writing), the consent of the person with the authority will be valid and there is no duty on the dentist to try and contact those with parental responsibility as well, unless there is reason to believe that the parent's view might differ.

Under section 3 of The Children Act 1989, a person who does not have parental responsibility for a particular child but has the care of that child may do what is reasonable in all circumstances for the purpose of safeguarding or promoting the child's welfare. Thus, a child who has fallen over in the playground and suffered trauma might be brought to the practice by a teacher when a parent cannot be contacted. It would be lawful for the dentist in this situation to provide treatment in the child's best interest, even if the teacher has not been given explicit authority to consent on behalf of the parents.

INCOMPETENT ADULTS

It is useful to deal with this group of patients separately, although in some ways the approach to obtaining consent is close to that of children. This group of patients lack capacity to consent in law by reason of lack of understanding due to mental illness, or by reason of unconsciousness. Nobody has the power to consent to treatment on behalf of an incompetent adult. It is a commonly held belief that consent can be obtained from a spouse, parent or near relative. This is not the case. Whilst it might be useful to seek to involve members of the family in deciding the best treatment for the patient, their consent or failure to provide it is not binding on the dentist.

Best interests

In English law, the lawfulness of invasive treatment given to incompetent adults is determined by reference to what is considered in their best interests. A dentist has a duty of care to judge what is in the patient's best interest and is legally accountable for this decision.

In deciding what is in the patient's best interest, the Bolam test would apply. The dentist must act in accordance with a responsible and competent body of relevant professional opinion in making decisions about treatment. In doing this, a dentist should consult another dentist when in doubt, and record any discussion in the records.

Another approach to treating this group of patients is to consider a *substituted judgement*. In this test, the decision maker acts as a proxy and makes a decision based on the patient's known views and values, with the intention that had the patient been mentally competent they would make the same judgement. This form of decision-making process has found some favour in the United States (in place of the 'best interests' test) but remains problematic in the UK.

FURTHER READING

Department of Health. Seeking consent: working with children. London: HMSO; 2001.

Department of Health. Reference guide to consent for examination or treatment. London: HMSO; 2001.

Grubb A, Laing JM. Principles of medical law. 2nd edn. Oxford: Oxford University Press; 2004.

Principles of patient consent. www.gdc-uk.org

Hockton A. The law of consent to medical treatment. London: Sweet and Maxwell; 2002.

REFERENCES

1 Dworkin R. Life's Dominion: An argument about Abortion and Euthanasia. London: Harper Collins; 1993.
2 St Georges Healthcare NHS Trust v. S [1983] 2 FLR 728 at 739C.
3 Re MB [1997] 2 FLR 426 at 432.
4 Lord Goff in Re F (Mental patient sterilisation) [1990] 2 AC 1.
5 Lord Donaldson in Re F [1992] AC 1 at 72.
6 Chatterton v. Gerson [1981] 1 All ER 257.
7 Appleton and Others v. Garrett [1997] 8 Med LR 75.
8 Department of Health. Reference guide to consent for examination or treatment. London: HMSO; 2001.
9 Ibid.
10 Principles of patient consent. London: GDC; May 2005.
11 Family Law Reform Act 1969. London: HMSO.
12 Gillick v. West Norfolk and Wisbech Area Health Authority [1986] 1 AC 112; 1985 3 All E.R. 402.
13 Re MB (An adult: medical treatment) [1997] 2 FCR 541.
14 Hope T, Savulescu J, Hendrick J. Medical ethics and law. Edinburgh: Churchill Livingstone; 2003.
15 Re C (adult: refusal of medical treatment) [1994] 1 All ER 819.
16 Kennedy I, Grubb A. Medical Law. 3rd edn. London: Butterworths; 2000; 753.
17 Re T (adult refusal of treatment) [1992] 4 All ER 640; [1992] 9 BMLR 46 (CA).
18 Sidaway v. Board of Governors of the Bethlem Royal Hospital [1985] AC 871.
19 Bolitho v. City and Hackney Health Authority [1988] AC 232.
20 Pearce v. United Bristol Healthcare Trust [1998] 48 BMLR 118 (CA).
21 Chester v. Afshar [2004] UK HL 41 (House of Lords).
22 NHS Litigation Authority. NHSLA risk alert: informed consent. Issue Number 4, November 2004 (www.nhsla.com).
23 Lingual nerve damage. Medical Protection Society UK Casebook 2004; 12(3): 21.
24 Patel AM. Appropriate consent and referral for general anaesthesia—a survey in the Paediatric Day Care Unit, Barnsley DGH NHS Trust, South Yorkshire. Br Dent J 2004; 196:275–277.
25 Mohamed Tahir MA, Mason C, Hind V. Informed consent: optimism versus reality. Br Dent J 2002; 193(4):221-224.
26 Reibl v. Hughes [1980] 114 DLR (3d) (Canada).
27 Lybert v. Warrington HA [1996] 7 Med LR 71.
28 Grubb A (ed). Principles of medical law. 2nd edn. Oxford: Oxford University Press; 2004; 319.
29 King J. Consent: the patients' view—a summary of findings from a study of patients' perceptions of their consent to dental care. Br Dent J 2001; 191:36–40.
30 Adewumi A, Hector MP, King JM. Children and informed consent: a study of children's perceptions and involvement in consent to dental treatment. Br Dent J 2001; 191:256–259.
31 Department of Health. Seeking consent: working with children. London: HMSO; 2001.
32 Hope T, Savulescu J, Hendrick J. Medical ethics and law: the core curriculum. Edinburgh: Churchill Livingstone; 2003; 139.
33 Re R (A minor) (Wardship: Medical treatment) [1992] 1 FLR 190 at 196.

Confidentiality

4

A uniformed police officer comes to the practice requesting the dental records for a patient he believes has been treated by the practice. He wants the records in connection with an assault. A solicitor writes to you requesting a dental report for a client, following a road traffic accident. A purse is stolen from a patient's coat hanging in the waiting room, and the only suspect is another patient. The victim of the theft wants the details of the suspect patient.

These are common problems faced by practitioners, the solutions to which are sometimes complex, sometimes surprising but all underpinned by common principles. Once these principles are understood, it becomes easier to approach issues of confidentiality in general dental practice.

The dentist–patient relationship is based on trust, and one of the most powerful expressions of this is the expectation that everything that takes place in the dental surgery will be kept confidential by the practice staff. However, this expectation is not an absolute one and exceptions do exist.

One of the most fundamental ethical obligations owed by a doctor to a patient is to respect the confidences of that patient. That this has long been a central premise in our approach to medicine can be seen from the fact that the Hippocratic oath states:

> 'Whatsoever things I see or hear concerning the life of men, in attendance on the sick or even apart therefrom, which ought not to be noised abroad, I will keep silence thereon, counting such things as sacred secrets.'[1]

In 1996, a British consultant neurologist discussed a teenage patient with suspected Creutzfeldt–Jakob disease during a television interview. He gave enough details for a newspaper to identify her, and her family was stalked for weeks by reporters. The General Medical Council carried out a full investigation, and whilst the doctor was eventually cleared of serious professional misconduct in respect of unnecessary breach of confidentiality, he was still criticised for his behaviour.[2]

In the context of this chapter, confidentiality is defined as the statutory and professional duty to safeguard personal information by preventing its improper disclosure. Personal information is defined as information about people which dentists and their teams learn in a professional capacity and from which individuals can be identified, either directly or indirectly. See Box 4.1 for GDC guidelines on dealing with patient confidentiality.

Confidentiality, as a human right, is protected by the Human Rights Act 1998. Article 8 of the European Convention on Human Rights provides:

1. Everyone has the right to respect for his private and family life, his home and his correspondence.
2. There shall be no interference by a public authority with the exercise of this right, except such as is in accordance with the law and is necessary in a democratic society in the interests of national security, public safety or the economic well being of the country, for the prevention of disorder or crime, for the protection

---

Box 4.1 GDC guidelines standards for dental professionals

- Treat information about patients as confidential and only use it for the purpose for which it is given.
- Prevent accidental disclosure or unauthorised access to confidential information by keeping information secure at all times.
- In exceptional circumstances, disclosure of confidential information without consent may be justified in the public or patient's interest. Seek appropriate advice before disclosing information on this basis.

of health or morals, or for the protection of the rights and freedoms of others.

When deciding whether a breach of Article 8 has occurred the court will decide whether the interferences are justified: a) in accordance with domestic UK law; b) there was a legitimate aim in breaching this right to privacy; and c) it was necessary in a democratic society.

This three-stage test was the basis of making a judgement in *Z* v. *Finland*,[3] which ruled on the confidentiality of Z's medical records which were disclosed in the course of an investigation into sexual assaults carried out by X, who was HIV-positive and married to Z, a Swedish national.

The Court had this to say:

'The Court will take into account that the protection of personal data, not least medical data, is of fundamental importance to a person's enjoyment of his or her right to respect for private and family life as guaranteed by Article 8 of the Convention. Respecting the confidentiality of health data is a vital principle in the legal systems of all the Contracting Parties of the Convention. It is crucial not only to respect the sense of privacy of a patient but also to preserve his or her confidence in the medical profession and in the health service in general.'

Since the case in question related to HIV infection, it is worth noting what the judges had to say, as this has direct relevance to general dental practice.

'The disclosure of such data [a person's HIV infection] may dramatically affect his or her private and family life, as well as social and employment situations, by exposing him or her to opprobrium and the risk of ostracism. For this reason it may also discourage persons from seeking diagnosis or treatment and thus undermine any preventive efforts by the community to contain the pandemic. The interest in protecting the confidentiality of such information will therefore weigh heavily in the balance in determining whether the interference was proportionate to the legitimate aim pursued. Such interferences cannot be compatible with Article 8 of the Convention unless justified by an overriding requirement in the public interest.'

Therefore, it would be hard to conceive of a situation in the context of general dental practice where the disclosure of such confidential information, such as the HIV status of a patient, would be in the interest of the public. However, the converse is not true, and HIV-positive and Hepatitis B/C-positive healthcare workers would be classed a risk to patients and therefore, by definition, the public. The issue surrounding the duty of confidentiality here is different, and one to which we will return later on.

DISCLOSURE OF CONFIDENTIAL INFORMATION ON ECONOMIC GROUNDS

Disclosure can be justified by Article 8(2) in certain circumstances other than those identified by *Z* v. *Finland*, where the grounds were 'preventing crime' and 'protecting the rights and freedoms of others'. In *MS* v. *Sweden*,[4] which also went to the European Court of Human Rights, medical records of MS were disclosed to the Social Insurance Office following her claim for compensation under the Industrial Injury Insurance Act in Sweden. The medical records from her doctor revealed much about her past history, and her claim for compensation was rejected by the Social Insurance Office on the grounds that her sick leave had not been caused by an industrial injury.

Here it was argued by MS that the information collected and stored at her doctor's surgery in connection with medical treatment should not have been passed on since this communication to another government department, albeit to assess her claim, served a different purpose and one to which she had not consented. In finding against her application, the court relied on the need to 'protect the economic well being of the country'. Since the other agencies which received the medical information were also under a similar duty to the doctor's clinic to treat the data as confidential, it was argued that the disclosure was limited in any case.

This has relevance in general practice in two specific areas. The first is the relationship of the Inland Revenue and patient records, and the second relates to patients waiving their rights to confidentiality, specifically in signing the NHS form FP17.

Inland revenue investigations

The Inland Revenue, in order to check the veracity of a dentist's accounts, is empowered under the Taxes Management Act 1970 (section 19a) to serve a notice requiring the dentist to

> '...produce to the officer such documents as are in the taxpayer's possession or power and as the officer may reasonably require for the purpose of determining whether, and if so, the extent to which (i) the return is incorrect or incomplete.'

Case law offers little confirmation whether the financial affairs between dentist and patient have the necessary quality of confidence about them, but the profession has commonly considered any information sought by the Inland Revenue from which patients' identity is ascertainable should be classified as confidential information.

As stated below, disclosure of confidential information without patient consent is permitted only when:

a. required by law and
b. when disclosure of the information is in the public's interest.

Disclosure required under (a) is under compulsion, therefore, and the duty of confidence is automatically overridden by the duty to comply with the law of the land (*Parry–Jones* v. *Law Society*[5] and *Hunter* v. *Mann*[6]). In the latter case, a doctor was compelled under section 168 of the Road Traffic Act 1972 to provide the name of a patient who was a dangerous driver.

The Human Rights Act (Article 8 in particular) confers qualified rights on the patient to have respect for their private lives, but disclosure is authorised where it is potentially for the economic well being of the country and could assist in the prevention of crime (tax fraud). Thus, the Human Rights Act actually confers legitimacy on the action of the Inland Revenue to pursue disclosure of patients' records.

Similarly, the Data Protection Act, whilst recognising that the dental records may contain sensitive data (as defined in section 2 of the Data Protection Act 1998), allows disclosure without consent of the patient if required by law or any enactments, by any rule of law or by order of a court. The Taxes Management Act 1970 is just such a rule of law and, therefore, the Data Protection Act offers no protection of the records from disclosures.

The Inland Revenue officers themselves are under their own duty of confidentiality and will in any case only request records as a last resort. Thus, if the Inland Revenue decided to conduct an enquiry under section 9A of the Taxes Management Act 1970 into the accuracy of a dentist's tax returns, a notice may be served (so long as certain notice formalities are complied with). Even if the dental records requested contain only one (or even no) valid entry necessary to check the accuracy of the tax return, a request for disclosures of the whole dental record, including the medical history, could be validly made.

A dental record is thus disclosable to the Inland Revenue. Defence organisations now suggest that financial transactions are kept separate from the treatment records in order to protect confidential information being disclosed in any tax investigation. Computer programmes are capable of doing this and, therefore, a request for a print-out with just the patient's name and details along with the financial transactions can be disclosed without fear of breaching patient confidentiality. The GDC has agreed in the past that, as a statutory body, it would expect dentists to comply with the law and assist government officials whose job it is to enforce the law.[7]

For manually kept records, a separate card/log for financial transactions should be kept. This card should carry both NHS and private financial transactions with dates of payments but no treatment details.

Patient declaration made by NHS patients

As part of the administration of an NHS course of treatment, a patient has to sign various forms, one of which is a claim form, an FP17 or PR (practice record) form. The FP17 manual claim form is sent to the payment agency (the Dental Practice Board) to confirm what treatment has been provided by the dentist and to enable payment to be claimed.

A claim can also be generated electronically by computer and transmitted to the Dental Practice Board by an EDI link, in which case the PR form remains in the practice as a record of the patient's attendance for treatment.

The declaration which the patient signs states:

'To enable the NHS to check I have a valid exemption and to prevent and detect fraud and incorrectness, I consent to the disclosure of relevant information from this form to and by the Dental Practice Board, Prescription Pricing Authority, NHS Counter Fraud and Security Management Service, Department for Work and Pensions and Local Authorities'.

The consent by the patient to disclose information is a very narrow one and relates only to the patient's status as either a patient who pays the full NHS charge or one who is claiming exemptions for dental charges which fall into several categories. The consent does not extend to confidential information on the dental records.

COMMON LAW OBLIGATION OF CONFIDENCE

The common law basis of confidence is based on the courts' examination of cases from the fields of contract, equity and property.

'The duty of confidence will arise from a transaction, often a contract, in which event the duty may arise by reason of either an express or an implied term of that contract.'

Lord Goff A-G *v.* Guardian Newspaper[8]

In addition to common law, there is also a statutory basis to the obligation of confidence such as Abortion Regulations 1991, NHS (Venereal Diseases) Regulations 1974 and the Health Act 1999.

In general the four classes of information that have traditionally been protected by law or whose use has been restricted by the enforcement of confidences are:

- personal information confided in the context of a professional relationship of trust
- trade secrets
- government information
- artistic and literary confidences.

SCOPE OF THE DUTY OF CONFIDENCE

'The doctor is under a duty not to disclose [voluntarily], without the consent of his patients, information, which he, the doctor, has gained in his professional capacity.'

Hunter *v.* Mann[9]

Thus the obligation extends to all information received by the clinician about the patient and would include reports from third parties. This information may come directly from the patient or the dentist's own consultation with the patient, or it may come from a third party in circumstances in which the third party knows of the dentist–patient relationship. This occurs commonly in referral letters. For example, a consultant to whom a general practitioner has referred will copy his letters to other specialists back to the GDP to keep them informed about treatment and investigations of the referred patient.

What does actually constitute a breach of confidence?

If confidential information is disclosed, does it have to be deliberate to be a breach of confidence? It has been argued that intention is not a factor, and even inadvertent disclosure of confidential information still constitutes a legal wrong.

In summary, the obligations in keeping confidences are these:[10]

- There is an important public interest in maintaining clinical confidentiality.
- That interest is so strong that the law imposes a duty on clinicians to maintain confidences.
- The duty to keep confidences is not an absolute—sometimes the public interest in disclosure may override it, or statute or the disclosure process in litigation requires it.

AUDIT AND THE USE OF ANONYMISED INFORMATION

Anonymised patient information is used for research, audit and quality assurance, and for management purposes in practices. It is also used for teaching purposes and in publications, and presented in a way that does not allow identification. There is an implicit assumption that in an anonymised form, there is no breach of patient confidences since the patient cannot be identified.

This issue was discussed in *R* v. *Department of Health* (ex parte Source Informatics Ltd).[11] In this case, Source Informatics was a data-collecting company seeking to persuade GPs and pharmacists to allow then to collect data as to the prescribing habits of GPs. They believed this information would be of commercial value to drug companies, and would provide useful data for those interested in monitoring prescribing patterns.

The proposal was that, with the consent of the GPs, the pharmacist (for a fee and using software provided by Source Informatics) would download onto disc the name of the GP and the identity and quantity of the drugs prescribed, but nothing which could identify the patient. The dispute arose because the Department of Health felt that anonymisation did not, in their view, remove the duty of confidence towards the patients who are the subject of the data, and argued that doctors involved in this scheme would be breaching patient confidentiality.

In making his conclusion, the judge argued that whilst the consultation leading to the prescription and the information on the prescription handed in to the pharmacist was confidential, it ceased to be so when it was anonymised and became purely statistical, carrying with it no information of a personal or private nature. Thus, no actual disclosure was made since the personal information could not be related to an individual patient and the patient's personal privacy was maintained.

Therefore, the key in processing personal information for use other than for the patient's direct treatment or diagnosis is to anonymise the data. In this context, a useful definition of personal information has been provided by Professor Raymond Wacks in his book *Personal information: privacy and the law*:[12]

> 'Personal information consists of those facts, communications, or opinions which relate to the individual and which it would be reasonable to expect him to regard as intimate or sensitive and therefore want to withhold or at least restrict their collection, use or circulation.'

More importantly, an essential element in any claim for breach of confidence is that the claimant should have suffered detriment and would not have if anonymity had been secured. The breach of confidence, even if it can be considered as such with anonymised information, could be acceptable if it was in the public interest, although in this case (*R v. Department of Health*) that was never argued.

CALDICOTT GUARDIANS

The Caldicott Committee was established by the Chief Medical Officer in England to review all patient-identifiable information that passes from NHS organisations to other NHS or non-NHS bodies for purposes other than direct care, medical research or where there is a statutory requirement for information. The purpose was to ensure that only the minimum necessary information is transferred in each case.

The report[13] summarised the responsibilities in six key principles:

1. Justify the purpose of using or transferring the information.
2. Patient-identifiable information should not be used unless it is absolutely necessary.
3. Use the minimum necessary patient-identifiable information.
4. Access to patient-identifiable information should be on a strict need-to-know basis.
5. Everyone in a team should know his or her own duties and responsibilities in relation to confidential information.
6. Understand and comply with the law.

Central to the implementation of this standard is the appointment of an individual with responsibility for taking this work forward and overseeing its continual development—the Caldicott guardian.

It is unlikely that any but the largest dental practices or groups would need to appoint their own Caldicott guardians. Dental practices are not NHS organisations and are unlikely ever to transfer information to non-NHS organisations. Any data transferred from practices is usually to the Dental Practice Board or in referral for specialist care.[14]

STATUTE PROTECTION

Two aspects of the Data Protection Act 1998 allow a practitioner holding dental records (as a data controller) to process that information for a number of 'legitimate' purposes.

> *Schedule 2 6(1) The processing is necessary for the purpose of legitimate interest pursued by the data controller or by the third party or parties to whom the data are disclosed, except where the processing is unwarranted in any particular case by reason of prejudice to the rights and freedoms or legitimate interests of the data subject.*

This condition allows disclosure for the purposes of research, financial accounting, management, audit, preventing fraud within the NHS, for maintaining professional standards or pursuing legal action against another, or defending action brought against an NHS body.[15]

The second protection for audit comes from Schedule 3, paragraph 8 of the Data Protection Act:

> 8(1) the processing is necessary for medical purposes and is undertaken by—
> a) A health professional, or
> b) A person who in the circumstances owes a duty of confidentiality which is equivalent to that which would arise if that person were a health professional
>
> (2) In this paragraph 'medical purposes' includes the purposes of preventative medicine, medical diagnosis, medical research, the provision of care and the management of healthcare services.

NHS/HEALTH AUTHORITY RIGHTS OF ACCESS TO CONFIDENTIAL INFORMATION

General dental practitioners who provide NHS services have a contract with their primary care trust (PCT) in England and Wales. This will grant the PCTs rights of access to dental records that will by definition contain confidential information. By the nature of the contract, which is also a financial one, the PCTs will also have access to financial and administrative records including appointment schedules.

The Healthcare Commission also has statutory access granted to it through the Health and Social Care Act 2003, and this is discussed later.

The Audit Commissions Act 1998 contains provisions for dealing with access to premises, information and data in an NHS context. These provisions allow the Audit Commissions to

- Require a person holding or accountable for any such document to give him such information and explanation as he thinks necessary for the purposes of his functions under the Act and
- If necessary, require the person to attend before him in person to give the information or explanation or to produce the document.

Failure to comply is an offence.

CONFIDENTIAL INFORMATION IN THE PRACTICE ENVIRONMENT

The duty of confidentiality owed to patients also extends to the staff in a dental practice. This should be made clear both in training new members of staff and in contracts, with the added support of a written confidentiality policy and clause inserted into the staff employment contracts.

It is a valid assumption that patients will be aware that disclosure of confidential information will occur within the healthcare team, so that typing of referral letters and all administration duties will involve the handling of dental records. The same is not necessarily true of information discussed with other dentists outside the practice team, as may occur in peer review meetings, case discussions or treatment planning meetings. Therefore, consent should be sought from patients before discussing personal information with individuals not directly involved in their clinical care, or with team members whose involvement might not be readily apparent, such as a laboratory technician.

EXAMINATIONS ON BEHALF OF A THIRD PARTY

Dentists may sometimes obtain confidential information through examination of a patient at the behest of another. This may be in the context of an insurance company, or an employer assessing dental fitness either prior to employment or a posting abroad. This situation also may occur in the Armed Forces.

In these cases, any personal information will have the necessary quality of confidence, but the scope of the duty of confidence owed to the patient is limited by the circumstances in which it is confided. In other words, the patient ought to know, because of the circumstances of the examination, that any information will be conveyed to the employer or insurance company in the dentist's report.

Nevertheless, it is important that the patient has been told at the earliest opportunity about the purpose of the examination, the extent of the information to be disclosed and the fact that relevant information cannot be concealed or withheld. It is important also to obtain or have seen written consent to the disclosure from the patient, or a person properly authorised to act on the patient's behalf.

In compiling the report, include only factual information you can substantiate, and in all circumstances you should check whether the patient wishes to see the report (unless the patient has clearly and specifically stated a wish not to do so).[16]

The duty of confidentiality can be breached in only two circumstances:

1. with the consent of the patient
2. in the public interest to protect others from risk of death or serious harm.

Thus, there is a balance to be judged by the clinician between the dual obligation of maintaining confidentiality and breaching it in the public interest. An important safeguard with respect to this disclosure of information is that the 'receivers' of any confidential information are bound by a legal duty of confidence, regardless of their professional obligations. This would apply equally to the person who types the report and the employees of the insurance company that receive the report as it would do to PCT staff who handle dental records and complaints.

CHILDREN AND ISSUES OF CONFIDENTIALITY

There is no doubt that a dentist owes a child patient a duty of confidentiality, and this has been upheld in a number of cases.[17,18] However, in keeping with the law of consent, the competence of the child and capacity to understand and form a relationship in confidence is significant. Therefore, when the child is incompetent to form a relationship of confidentiality, the dentist is obliged to disclose the information to the parent. The law's paramount concern is the welfare of the child, and in most cases the welfare of the child is best served by the parents knowing all the dental information available to allow them to make a decision or assist in care.

Children at risk

Where a child lacks the capacity to consent to treatment and also to enter into a confidential relationship, the law would expect the dentist to act in the child's best interest. If the dentist believes the child to be a victim of neglect or physical, sexual or emotional abuse, the information should be given promptly to an appropriate responsible person or statutory agency, where the clinician believes the disclosure is in the patient's best interests. If, on balance, the dentist believes the child is at risk from the parent, then they can legitimately disclose the information to someone else.

Where a child has capacity both to consent to treatment and enter into a confidential relationship, obligations of confidence exist and are no different to those owed to an adult. Here a breach of duty of confidence may be justified if it is made in the public interest or the patient's best interests. In either case, the dentist will need to be able to justify the disclosure.

MODIFICATION OF THE DUTY OF CONFIDENCE

As we have seen above in relation to children, the legal duty of maintaining patient confidentiality is not an absolute one and may be subject to exceptions.

There are three main exceptions:

1. where consent by the patient has been given to allow disclosure
2. in the public interest
3. where the law compels disclosure.

Consent to allow disclosure

When a patient gives consent, the dentist is no longer under an obligation to keep the confidence. As for patients consenting for treatment, the consent requires that the patient:

- has the capacity to decide
- has sufficient information to make a decision
- is acting voluntarily with no undue influence exerted on them.

In reality, the stumbling block will be how much information constitutes a sufficient amount. The ethical requirement, as well as the legal standards, would anticipate that the patient is informed in a broad way about what is to be disclosed and for what purposes that disclosed information might be used. Most consent is *express* but could also be contractual where information, particularly financial, is used for administrative and probity reasons (where taxpayer's money is involved in NHS treatment). If there is a practice of disclosure in these circumstances, for the patient's *implied* consent to be valid, the patient must at least be aware of the practice, be given an opportunity to object and not do so.

Express consent to disclose confidential information would not be required in the context of a receptionist typing referral letters, or to a specialist to whom the patient has agreed to be referred. Dentists cannot treat patients safely nor provide the continuity of care without having the relevant information about the patient's condition and medical history.[19]

Public interest

There are some occasions where the need to disclose confidential information with or without the patient's consent is done in the public interest and outweighs the public interest in protecting the individual's right to confidence. Therefore, there is a judgement to be made in balancing the two interests and deciding which is favoured.

In the context of medical confidences, the public interest in preserving confidences comes about because of the very nature of the dentist–patient relationship. Take for example a diagnosis of HIV in the case history below.

Kennedy and Grubb[21] usefully categorise the types of situation where public interest may used

in justifying disclosures of confidential information:

1. where there is a danger to the health or safety of others
2. where a crime is to be prevented or detected
3. where there is a need for research, teaching or management purposes.

Danger to the health or safety of others

There is a clear need to balance the needs of the individual against the needs of the public, and in the case of *W* v. *Edgell*[22] (below) these came head to head.

Thus, it can be seen that the law recognises an important public interest in maintaining professional duties of confidence, but the law treats such duties not as absolutes. They are liable to be overridden where there is held to be a stronger public interest in disclosure. In this case, on balance, it was felt that Dr Edgell was right to make the disclosure. He did so in accordance with law, and it was necessary in the interest of public safety and the prevention of crime.

X v. *Y*[20]

In February 1987, one or more employees of the plaintiffs, a health authority, supplied the first defendant, a reporter on a national newspaper owned and published by the second defendants, with information obtained from hospital records which identified two doctors who were carrying on general practice despite having contracted the disease AIDS.

The second defendants made one or more payments of £100 for the information. On 28 February, the plaintiffs (the doctors) obtained an order restraining the defendants from 'publishing…or making any use whatsoever of any confidential information' which was the property of the plaintiffs and contained in their hospital records. On 15 March, the second defendants published an article written by the first defendant, under the headline 'Scandal of Docs with AIDS', which implied that there were doctors in Britain who were continuing to practise despite having contracted AIDS, and that the Department of Health and Social Security wished to suppress that fact.

The defendants intended to publish a further article identifying the doctors. The plaintiffs sought: (i) an injunction restraining the defendants from publishing the identity of the two doctors; (ii) disclosure by the defendants of their sources. The question arose whether the second defendants were justified in the public interest in publishing and using the information disclosed to the first defendant.

In giving judgement on this point, Justice Rose was clear why patients, in this case who happened to be doctors, have a need to be sure confidential information is kept private.

'If it [confidential information] is breached, or if the patients have grounds for believing that it may be or has been breached they will be reluctant to come forward for and continue with treatment, and in particular counselling…If treatment is not provided or continued, the individual will be deprived of its benefit and the public are likely to suffer from an increase in the rate of spread of the disease. The preservation of confidentiality is therefore in the public interest.'

Whilst the judge recognised the very important public interest in the freedom of the press and that there was some public interest in knowing who the doctors were, he concluded that 'those public interests are substantially outweighed when measured against the public interests in relation to loyalty and confidentiality, both generally and with particular reference to AIDS patients' hospital records.'

He therefore granted an injunction preventing the naming of the doctors.

W v. Edgell

This case related to W, a patient who was detained in a secure hospital without time limit as a potential threat to public safety after he shot and killed five people and wounded two others. Ten years after he had been first detained he applied to a Mental Health Review Tribunal (MHRT) to be discharged. His responsible medical officer supported the application, but this was opposed by the Government acting through the Secretary of State.

In order to assist his case, W's solicitors engaged Dr. Edgell, a consultant psychiatrist, to examine their client W and report on his mental condition. In the event, Dr. Edgell strongly opposed the transfer, confirming the patient's continued interest in firearms and explosives.

Dr. Edgell sent the report to W's solicitors, who withdrew the application to the MHRT to have their client discharged. Neither the tribunal nor the hospital looking after W received the report, but Dr. Edgell was concerned that in the patient's interest, for treatment and also the public's wider protection, the report should be seen by other parties. W discovered the report was disclosed and issued a writ against Edgell and the recipients of the report, seeking an injunction to restrain them from using or disclosing the report further.

In making his judgement, Stephen Brown J pointed to the General Medical Council guidance as being particularly relevant:

81(b) Confidential information may be shared with other registered medical practitioners who participate in or assume responsibility for clinical management of the patient.

(g) Rarely, disclosure may be justified on the ground that it is in the public interest which, in certain circumstances such as, for example, investigation by the police of a grave or very serious crime, might override the doctor's duty to maintain his patient's confidence.

82. Whatever the circumstances, a doctor must always be prepared to justify his action if he has disclosed confidential information. If a doctor is in doubt whether any of the exceptions mentioned above would justify him in disclosing information in a particular situation he will be wise to seek advice from a medical defence society or professional organisation.

If a confidence is to be breached, what guidance is there regarding the limit of the extent of information that can be disclosed?

This can be summarised as follows:

1. **Need to know limitation.** Disclosure may only be made to those whom it is necessary to tell so as to protect the public interest. In this case this is done without consent 'where a failure to do so may expose the patient or others to a risk of death or serious harm'.[23] However, it is normal to seek consent to disclosure when at all possible.
2. **The risk must be real.**
3. **Where there is a danger of physical harm.** This may include parents or relatives abusing their children, and dental practitioners may recognise oro-facial signs of abuse or be presented with unexplained injuries or bite marks. This may also include infectious diseases such as HIV and AIDS.

Managing issues of confidentiality with HIV/AIDS patients

The potential for patients to be stigmatised by having HIV and AIDS, and the impact it may have on family life and employment, makes this issue particularly important when it comes to confidentiality. General dental practitioners are unlikely to make a definite diagnosis of AIDS or HIV in their practices, but they may be given the information in a medical history questionnaire. That information is naturally confidential, but you may disclose information to a known sexual contact of a patient with HIV where you have reason to think that the patient has not informed that person and cannot be persuaded to do so. In such circumstances, you should tell the patient before you make the disclosure, and you must be prepared to justify that decision.[24]

Where you have made a referral and a diagnosis has been made, it is likely that the patient would have been counselled about the nature of the disease and its social and occupational implications. Your duty in these circumstances would be to ensure that other healthcare workers, such as the patient's GP, are also informed.

The infected person may of course be another dentist or other healthcare worker (HCW), but they are entitled to receive the same rights of confidentiality as any patient seeking or receiving medical care.

In its guidance, the Department of Health reiterates the importance of ensuring every effort is made to avoid disclosure of the infected worker's identity, or information which would allow deductive disclosure. This should include the use of a media injunction as necessary to prevent publication or other disclosure of a worker's identity.

However, it confirms that the duty of confidentiality is not absolute. Legally, the identity of infected individuals may be disclosed with their consent, or without in exceptional circumstances where it is considered necessary for the purpose of treatment, or prevention of spread of infection.[25]

The GDC have addressed this situation in 'Standards for Dental Professionals' (see Appendix 6).

Fitness to practise issues

Patient records or other patient information may be needed by a statutory regulatory body, such as the General Dental Council, for investigation into a health professional's fitness to practise. The patient's consent must be sought before disclosing identifiable information whenever practicable. The Dentist Act 1984 gives the GDC the power to require dentists to supply any document or information which appears relevant to the discharge of the GDC functions, provided that disclosure is not prohibited by other legislation.

Prevention or detection of crime

Where prevention or detection of crime may require the disclosure of confidential information there are some circumstances when that disclosure may be justifiable. The problem is what constitutes a crime. The GMC defines crimes as having to be 'serious', and that they 'will put someone at risk of death or serious harm, and will usually be crimes against the person, such as abuse of children'.

As in all issues of confidentiality, the decision to disclose confidential information to the police, for example, will depend on balancing the public interest in favour of it or against it. The less serious the crime, the less likely the patient's confidentiality should be breached.

In an attempt to reduce fraud and corruption in the NHS, the Government established the NHS Counter Fraud and Security Management Service (CFSMS) as a special health authority in 2003 following the success of the NHS Counter Fraud service which was established in September 1998. In the longer term, the CFSMS will become part of the new Business Services Authority (BSA). The CFSMS, in order to carry out their investigations, will always require access to relevant documents and records, including clinical records and data. They often work with the police and make use of their powers of search and arrest. The CFSMS are currently looking for more powers to provide access rights to information to enable the NHS counter fraud specialists to deal themselves with the majority of their cases without involving the police.

Teaching, research and clinical audit

There are a number of situations where confidential material obtained in practice may be used for teaching purposes. Case histories, including radiographs and photographs, may be used in small group teaching or in presentations, and in this case express consent must be obtained if it is possible that the patient can be identified. If the information is being used for exam purposes, then written consent must be obtained. Where records have been anonymised by the dentist or a member of the healthcare team, the patient's express consent is not required. If a general practice is utilised for hands-on teaching purposes for other dentists, the consent of the patient must be obtained to enable non-treating clinicians to view confidential information, including radiographs and study casts.

Clinical audit is an important aspect of ensuring the delivery of high quality care in general dental practice. All NHS dentists have a duty to participate in clinical audit. It is usual where an internal audit is to be carried out by the dental team that provided the care that identifiable information can be shared by the team as long as the patients have been informed that their data may be disclosed for clinical audit. Arguably, unless outside members of the treating team are involved in processing the raw data (such as other dentists or nurses), the existing obligation of confidentiality will exist and no further consent is required. It may be appropriate to inform patients that audit does takes place, preferably in a welcome letter or pack, or practical information leaflet supplied to patients.

Where data are being shared outside of the practice, care must be taken to anonymise any data so that the patient cannot be identified, even inadvertently.

Management and NHS administrative purposes

Where provision of NHS dental services is being administered locally through primary care trusts, there is greater potential for disclosure of confidential information relating to patient care. Patient details are related directly to the provision of treatment for the purposes of payment, and it is therefore impractical to anonymise this information before it leaves the practice. The same applies when records are requested by health authority staff to verify payments or the provision of treatment.

The basis of this disclosure is likely to be *implied* consent from the patient since the NHS would not be able to carry out its functions or fulfil its obligations to the tax payer with respect to the probity of payments made to practices for dental treatment. Here the public interest approach of allowing disclosure enables this to be legally justified on the basis of protecting the 'economic well being of the country', as determined in *MS* v. *Sweden* (above).

More specifically the patient when signing certain NHS forms allows for the disclosure quite clearly (see above).

Statutory requirements to disclose

There are a number of statutory provisions that create a legal duty to disclose information relating to patients where breach under certain circumstances would be a criminal offence. Some of these will not impact on the work of a general dental practitioner, such as the Abortion Regulations 1991 and The National Health Services (Venereal Diseases) Regulations 1974.

The Public Health (Control of Disease) Act 1984 and the Public Heath (Infectious Diseases Regulations) 1998 similarly relate to diseases unlikely to be encountered by a GDP, but the effect of them is to make certain diseases or food poisoning cases notifiable by the doctor, where the patient's name, age and address are sent to the appropriate local office.

The Coroners Act allows coroners access to records in the course of investigating the death of a person. The coroner has powers to compel disclosure of information relevant to an inquiry, including dental records of the deceased. Where a police officer is acting with the coroner's authority, the deceased patient's records should be disclosed as requested. This occurs when forensic dental identification may be required in a body that cannot be identified by any other means (e.g. badly decomposed bodies, or those recovered after a flood, drowning, fire or other accident).

Police inquiry

The Police and Criminal Evidence Act 1984 (PACE) gives the police access to dental records deemed 'excluded material' only on application to a circuit judge. The duty of confidence rests with the holder of the personal records, where the personal records are 'documentary and other records concerning an individual (whether living or dead) who can be identified from them and relating to … his physical or mental heath'.

The police do not have an inherent right of access to confidential dental records, and a dentist is only obliged to provide this if the police have a court order or search warrant. If the police ask for records or the release of personal patient information, the first step would be to obtain the consent of the patient. If obtaining consent is impossible, or if it would be impractical or unreasonable to do so, then any decision about disclosing information must be one that the dentist is prepared to justify.

The provisions of PACE deal with access by the police and do not stop a dentist voluntarily disclosing the records, provided this would be a justified breach of confidence (e.g. in the public interest). Equally, where a dentist believes that he has an overriding duty of confidence to the patient and there can be no justification for the police requesting access to the records, the dentist is entitled to ask the police to obtain an order from a judge forcing him to do so. The dentist may wish to make representation to the circuit judge that an order should not be made.

R v. *Singleton* (below) confirms the seriousness with which statute law regards the protection of such material and the duty of confidence placed on a dentist even in the face of an allegation of murder.

Health and Social Care Act 2003

The Commission of Healthcare Audit and Improvement (CHAI) (now known as The Healthcare

R v. Singleton[26]

Singleton was charged with murder. After his arrest he was asked by the police to provide a sample of tooth marks because the victim had marks on her chin which were thought to have been made by a human bite. He refused, but his dentist voluntarily gave his dental records to the police.

Singleton sought at his trial to have the dental evidence excluded on the grounds that it was excluded material within the terms of section 11 of the Police and Criminal Evidence Act 1984, and as such could only be disclosed to the police by means of an application to a circuit judge under section 9 and paragraph 3 of Schedule 1 to the 1984 Act. The judge ruled that the evidence was admissible and the appellant was convicted. In the Appeal hearing, the judge noted that, had Singleton's dentist refused to disclose the records which included the study models, the police would not have been successful on an application for access under PACE and the trial against Singleton for murder could have failed.

Commission) has authority to enter and inspect dental practices providing NHS services and to take copies of documents including patient records. The way in which it obtains, handles, uses and discloses this confidential personal information is set out in its Code of Practice on access to personal information (www.healthcarecommission.org.uk).

The Act (under section 67) allows an authorised person to inspect, take copies of and remove from the premises any documents or records (including personal records). The authorised person can interview in private any person working at the premises, any person receiving healthcare there who consents to be interviewed, and make any other examination into the state and management of the premises and treatment of persons receiving healthcare there. The Act also allows access to computer records. It is a criminal offence to obstruct, without reasonable excuse, any authorised person carrying out their duties under this legislation.

CONFIDENTIALITY IN PRACTICE

Most breaches of confidentiality are inadvertent. Being alert to the issues of confidentiality means looking at the practice environment and the management systems carefully and establishing protocols with confidentiality in mind.

Reception

It is often difficult and indeed impractical to separate the waiting area from the reception and appointment booking area in general practice. This means that other patients can overhear conversations between the receptionist and a patient at the desk or on the phone. Receptionists need to be mindful of this, and certainly when speaking to patients over the phone they should avoid the broadcasting of identifiers such as name and address where possible.

The basic problem with a telephone call is that you do not know who is on the other end. You may have breached confidentiality simply by saying: 'Could I speak to Miss Jones, this is High Street Dental Practice here'. There are circumstances in which letting a third party know a dentist is calling them could be embarrassing, and it may be safer to identify yourself once it can be confirmed that the patient is on the other end of the line.

Caution must be exercised particularly when outstanding accounts or bad debts are being pursued, either by telephone from the practice or by post. In the latter case, marking any correspondence 'Private and Confidential' is important. Similarly, staff should be careful about discussing treatment or financial transactions with other members of a patient's family without the consent of the patient.

Patients often phone up to check their appointment times, or to cancel and make new ones. It is important to be certain that you are actually talking to the patient, and asking them to confirm their date of birth and address/phone number will assist this process.

Schools and employers may also telephone to confirm attendance of pupils or employees at the dentist. This is confidential information, and the patient's consent should always be sought before disclosing such information.

Relatives or partners also phone about appointments and are often given information about times and dates of treatment. This is, strictly speaking, a breach of confidentiality, and whilst it is important that your staff do not appear overly officious, the exigencies of confidentiality need to be recognised in a pragmatic but legal way.

Patients' records should not be left visible on the reception desk, and the computer screen should be angled away from patients or filtered with unidirectional screens so that appointments and confidential information relating to other patients cannot be viewed.

Treatment rooms

Whilst it might be appropriate for a whole family of children to be seen together, husbands and wives or other couples may not necessarily wish to be invited in to the treatment room together, as private and confidential information may need to be discussed. If work placement students or dental students are allowed to sit in during patient examinations, the duty of confidentiality must be made clear to them or any third party that has access to sensitive, personal data. Third parties present in a consultation must be introduced to the patient on arrival, and the patient informed of their status and why they are sitting in. The patient should be allowed to decline consent to allow the third party to be present but must not be made to feel that treatment will be affected in any way by declining.

SOME INTERESTING CASES

The following situations have all arisen in general dental practice, and an advisor at a defence organisation has been asked for advice. Having read this chapter you should be able to offer an answer.

Case 1
A 15-year-old orthodontic patient has an appointment for the dentist to adjust her fixed orthodontic appliance. The mother has phoned the practice saying she has listed her as missing but knows she has gone off with an older man. The mother wants the dentist to call the police when she arrives for her appointment. If he telephones the police he will be breaching her confidentiality. Is he allowed to do this without her consent?

Case 2
An appointment card for a dental appointment is found at the scene of a burglary. There is no patient's name on the card but there is a date and time on the card which also has the dentist's practice details. The police telephone the practice requesting the name and details of the patient whose appointment it is, in order to investigate a non-violent burglary.

Case 3
A regular patient's car is damaged in the practice car park by another car bumping into it, scratching the whole of one wing. She knows there was only one other car in the car park—a blue car—and there are blue flecks of paint on her own white car. She wants to know the name and address of the other patient whose car it is so she can claim on insurance. Can the practice disclose this information?

Case 4
A patient has attended the practice having had a number of drinks for lunch. He drove to the practice. After the appointment the dentist has asked the patient to leave the car behind till he sobers up, but the patient has declined this advice and driven off when potentially over the limit. Should she have done more to stop him, and can she inform the police?

Case 5
The dentist thinks the patient for whom he has planned an extraction is an alcoholic. He is concerned about the possibility of severe bleeding due to impaired liver function. When invited to do so, the patient's general medical practitioner will not disclose anything about his patient's medical history without the patient's consent. The patient himself denies being a drinker and will not disclose anything adverse about his medical history, saying he is fit and healthy. Does the medical GP have a right to withhold the information which may be of relevance to the dentist in the management of their joint patient?

FURTHER READING

Department of Health. Confidentiality: NHS Code of Practice. HMSO; 2003.(www.doh.gov.uk)

Foster C, Peacock N. Clinical Confidentiality. Sudbury: Monitor Press; 2000.

General Medical Council. Confidentiality: protecting and providing information. Manchester: General Medical Council; 2000.

Panting G, Hegan T. 1998 Data Protection Act simplified. Leeds: Medical Protection Society; 2000.

REFERENCES

1 Kennedy I, Grubb A. Medical Law. 3rd edn. London: Butterworths; 2000; 753.

2 McTigue A, Williams S. Have confidence in confidence alone. Casebook (Medical Protection Society) 2003; 4:8-10.

3 Z v. Finland [1997] 25 EHRR 371 (EctHR).

4 MS v. Sweden [1997] 45 BMLR 133 (EctHR).

5 Parry–Jones v. Law Society [1968] 1 All ER 177; [1969] 1 Ch 1.

6 Hunter v. Mann [1974] 2 Al ER 414; QB 767.

7 Correspondence from MH Ridler, GDC Fitness to Practise Director, March 2000.

8 Lord Goff A-G v. Guardian Newspaper (No 2)[1990] 1 AC 109 (the 'Spycatcher' case).

9 Hunter v. Mann [1974] QB 767.

10 Foster C, Peacock N. Clinical Confidentiality. Sudbury: Monitor Press; 2000.

11 R v. Department of Health, ex parte Source Informatics Ltd [1999] 52 BMLR 65 CA.

12 Wacks R. Personal information: privacy and the law. Oxford: Clarendon Press; 1989.

13 Department of Health, Caldicott Committee. Report on the review of patient-identifiable information. London: HMSO; 1997.

14 Caldicott guardians and questionnaires. BDA News 2002; 14(7):25.

15 Kennedy I, Grubb A. Medical Law. 3rd edn. London: Butterworths; 2000.

16 General Medical Council. Confidentiality: protecting and providing information. Manchester: General Medical Council; 2000.

17 Re C (a minor) (wardships: medical treatment) [1989] 2 All ER 791 (CA).

18 Re Z (a minor) (freedom of publication) [1995] 4 All ER 961 (CA).

19 General Medical Council. Confidentiality: protecting and providing information. Manchester: General Medical Council; 2000.

20 X v. Y [1988] 2 All ER 648; [1987] 3 BMLR 1 (QBD).

21 Kennedy I, Grubb A. Medical Law. 3rd edn. London: Butterworths; 2000; 753.

22 W v. Edgell [1990] 1 All ER 835; 4 BMLR 96 (CA).

23 General Medical Council. Confidentiality: protecting and providing information. Manchester: General Medical Council; 2000.

24 General Medical Council. Serious communicable diseases. General Medical Council; 1997 (http://www.gmc-uk.org/standards).

25 Department of Health. AIDS/HIV infected healthcare workers: guidance on the management of infected healthcare workers and patient notification. Department of Health; 1999.

26 R v. Singleton [1995] 1 Cr App Rep 431 (CA).

Clinical negligence

5

A number of studies[1] have highlighted that the fear of litigation in general dental practice ranks high amongst potential causes of stress to dentists. This real or imagined threat of being 'sued' has been fuelled by a number of factors. Foremost amongst these are increased patient expectations and a greater desire for patients to retain their teeth for life. The rise of aesthetic dentistry, with white straight teeth being equated with success and associated with media stars, is an important driver in this increasing consumerism, which is in part being driven by dentists themselves.

Only a small proportion of dental treatment results in patient complaints, and these are due mainly to inadequate dental care and unrealistic expectations, or a combination of the two. Patients expect more now in terms of both the information they are provided about their oral health and the longevity of the restorations that are placed in their mouths. When something goes wrong, they expect an explanation for it and, increasingly, compensation.

The defence organisations (Medical Defence Union, Medical Protection Society) reported a doubling of the frequency of claims between 1983 and 1987 alone.[2] In the dental claims unit of Dental Protection, claims have gone up from 550 in 1996 to 1180 in 2002. The same exponential rise has been seen in the number of complaints made by patients about the service and treatment that they received from dentists. In 2002, information from Dental Protection confirmed that dentists in the UK had the highest claims frequency in the world—that is, a dentist was more likely to be sued in the UK than in any other country in the world, including the USA.

Mistakes are costly. A recent analysis of incidents in the NHS generally has suggested that between 314 000 and 1.4 million NHS patients are harmed every year, and the report suggests that half of these mishaps (including surgical mistakes, hospital-acquired infections and prescribing errors) could have been avoided. The study also estimated that the mistakes cost the NHS £2 billion for the extra time patients needed to stay in hospital, on top of the clinical negligence costs running at more than £500 million a year.[3]

It is arguable whether this rise in claims reflects a declining standard of healthcare or an increasing awareness by patients of their rights, fuelled by almost daily media coverage of claims for compensation.

In this climate of litigation there is a natural tendency to practise 'defensive dentistry', in which clinical practice is altered to provide the 'safest' treatment. Such treatment may not necessarily be in the patient's best interest but provided on the basis that the chances of something going wrong and resulting in a lawsuit are reduced. This phenomenon is more common in medicine and can account for changes in practice, such as the increased provision of Caesarean section deliveries in obstetrics due to the higher incidence of complications in natural deliveries. Up to 28% of all births in some trusts may have less to do with women choosing an operation, and more to do with doctors' anxieties about being sued.[4]

The government is fully aware of the prevailing climate and the burdens it places on society and the taxpayer. In a document in response to a Better Regulation Task Force report, it said 'the government is determined to scotch any suggestion of a developing "compensation culture" where people believe that they can seek compensation for any misfortune that befalls them, even if no one else is to blame. This misconception undermines personal responsibility and respect for the law and creates unnecessary burdens through an exaggerated fear of litigation'.[5]

It is not all bad news; there is still an enormous amount of trust in the dental profession, with some 86% expressing a fair or great deal of confidence in their dentist.[6] In 2003–2004, figures from the Governments Compensation Recovery Unit (CRU), which collates information from all insurers (general accident and personal injury), showed a 60 000 drop in the number of claims from the previous year.

WHAT IS CLINICAL NEGLIGENCE?

In common everyday usage, 'negligence' has the well-recognised inference of 'carelessness' or lack of proper care and attention. It is used fairly loosely by patients, who may accuse their dentist of acting negligently, but in law it has a very specific meaning. Negligence is not merely making a mistake or something occurring accidentally. For a patient to be successful in a claim for negligence against a dentist, three essential features must be present and proved:

1. that a duty of care is owed by the dentist to the patient
2. there was breach of duty of care in failing to reach the standard of care expected
3. the patient suffered harm/losses as a result (causation) and that harm was foreseeable.

Clinical negligence is part of the general law of tort, where *tort* derives from the Latin for wrested, wrung or crooked. The word 'tort' is especially used to signify a civil, as opposed to criminal, wrong which is independent of a breach of contract or a crime. Examples of this class of action would be libel and trespass, and the intention in clinical negligence is primarily concerned with compensating patients who have suffered harm as a result of breaches of duties imposed by law. The sum of money paid (quantum) clearly cannot replace lost health or natural teeth, but the objective is to try and put the patient (claimant) in the same position as he or she would have been had the negligence never occurred.

DUTY OF CARE

'Duty of care' is the first hurdle a claimant has to surmount before an action in negligence can be commenced. In civil claims not involving a healthcare professional this is not always easy, as it must be shown that a duty of care was owed by that person to the claimant. The test that has come to be regarded as the 'neighbour' principle found its origins in Lord Atkins's judgement in *Donoghue* v. *Stevenson*.[7]

'Who then in law is my neighbour? Persons who are so closely and directly affected by my act that I ought reasonably to have them in contemplation as being so affected when directing my mind to the acts or omissions which are called in question.'

In this case, Mrs Donoghue visited a café where her friend bought a bottle of ginger beer to make a ginger beer float. The bottle of ginger beer was poured over the ice cream and consumed by Mrs Donoghue. The unnamed friend was later casually examining the opaque bottle when she discovered the remains of a decomposing snail. Having already drunk some, Mrs Donoghue suffered severe gastroenteritis and nervous shock. The problem for the House of Lords was that Mrs Donoghue was not the purchaser of the ginger beer and, therefore, had no contractual relationship with the seller. Instead, Mrs Donoghue pursued the manufacturer of the ginger beer. She won the case on the basis that negligence is a separate tort in its own right, and that negligence will arise when a duty is owed based on the neighbour principle.

Whilst this case confirmed that a manufacturer has a duty of care to all its potential customers, the notion of 'duty of care' has become increasingly flexible since this case in 1932. For example, a duty of care is owed by drivers to other road users and pedestrians, and a duty of care is owed not to cause nervous shock through careless acts, such as was highlighted in *McLoughlin* v. *O'Brian*[8] where a mother was compensated for nervous shock after seeing members of her family in various states of injury in the hospital casualty ward after a road traffic accident. Duty of care also extends to accountants or financial advisors who are entrusted not to cause economic loss through careless advice or transactions.

The case of *Caparo Industries plc* v. *Dickman*[9] confirmed that a duty of care arises when:

- it is foreseeable that the claimant would be affected by the acts and omissions of the defendant

- there is sufficient proximity between the parties
- the court considers that it would be fair, just and reasonable to impose a duty in all circumstances of the case.[10]

In general practice, as soon as a person is accepted by the dentist as a patient or examined, a duty of care exists. There is usually no argument raised where treatment or advice is provided, since a duty of care will normally automatically exist between the dentist and the patient.

In this context, a duty of care will also exist where advice is being sought at a social gathering, and so-called 'cocktail party' dental advice given in this situation, which is acted upon, may lead to a claim in negligence. Dentists are often asked for advice about clinical matters or invited to give opinions about a friend's on-going or past treatment. Without properly examining the person, it would be unwise to offer advice in this situation.

Emergencies

If a patient collapses in the dental practice, there will be a duty of care between the practice and the patient, and all reasonable attempts to care for the patient will be expected. What is a reasonable standard of care is something we will come to shortly, since the decision to stock a plethora of emergency drugs which you may not be competent to use is an important one and very relevant in such a situation.

However, there is currently no duty in UK law to act as a 'Good Samaritan',[11] but if a dentist or nurse does decide to assist someone who has collapsed (e.g. at a social gathering) the dentist assumes a duty of care not to make the victim's condition worse (*Capital Counties plc* v. *Hampshire CC*).[12]

In the context of out-of-hours emergency cover for NHS patients, this is currently provided by dentists themselves or through a rota but in future will be provided by the primary care trust in England and Wales, and they will have a statutory duty of care (Health and Social Care Act 2003).

For all patients, the GDC expects appropriate out-of-hours provision to be made, and for those arrangements to be made known to patients. What actually constitutes 'an emergency' which requires to be seen outside of normal working hours is the subject of some debate but has been defined by the Department of Health as a severe haemorrhage, a threatened airway or an overwhelming infection.[13] In the case of a patient in severe pain, some might argue there is a moral obligation to attend that patient, and perhaps even a professional obligation. However, moral obligations are not legal obligations and the two should not be confused.

BREACH OF DUTY

Once it has been established that the defendant dentist owes the claimant a duty of care, which as can be seen above is usually the case, the next issue is whether the dentist has provided an adequate standard of care in the situation. What then is the standard of care required? The answer quite simply is 'a reasonable standard', which poses the further question what is a reasonable standard and who is the arbiter of those standards.

The standard of care expected from a dentist is more than would be expected from the apocryphal 'man on the Clapham omnibus', which is the standard in the general law of negligence. The standard of care required by dentists in clinical negligence cases, which has become known as the 'Bolam test', is set out by McNair J in the case *Bolam* v. *Friern Hospital Management Committee*.[14]

> 'The test is the standard of the ordinary skilled man exercising and professing to have that special skill. A man need not possess the highest expert skill; it is well established in law that it is sufficient if he exercises the ordinary skill of the ordinary competent man exercising that particular art … a doctor is not guilty of negligence if he has acted in accordance with a practice accepted as proper by a responsible body of medical men skilled in that particular art (a doctor is not negligent if he is acting in accordance with such a practice, merely because there is a body of opinion which takes a contrary view).'

In this case, John Bolam, who was suffering from depression, was treated with electroconvulsive therapy (ECT). Because ECT can precipitate convulsive movements, muscle relaxants can be given or the patient restrained to avoid bone fractures and dislocations. Unfortunately, despite nurses positioned either side of him during the treatment, Bolam suffered bilateral hip fractures. The claimant alleged that the defendants were negligent in failing to administer muscle relaxants, did not provide adequate restraint and failed to warn him of the possible risks prior to treatment.

The experts on both sides agreed that there was a responsible body of opinion that would not administer muscle relaxants in ECT, and that excessive restraint could in fact lead to greater risk of injury. Therefore, there were two schools of opinion in the matter.

Since 1957, the Bolam test has been the basis upon which the standard of dental treatment has been judged in respect to claims of negligence. It is based on what a peer group of other dentists would do or not do in similar circumstances at the time in question.

A look at two cases of endodontic instrument fracture (below) illustrates this point.[15] Endodontic instrument fracture can happen to anyone—even specialists—but it is the action of the dentist subsequent to the event that will often determine whether there was any negligent conduct involved.

Since it may be many years later that a claim is brought to court, the standard expected would pertain to the time of treatment and not to some higher standards or guidelines that came about later. For example, the general usage of CPITN or BPE scores did not occur in general practice till the late 1980s, and therefore in a claim for failure to diagnose periodontal disease there should be no expectation that a practitioner would have routinely used this method to screen patients before this time.

Clinical judgement and differences in opinion

There is usually more than one way to provide treatment in any given situation, and the law recognises that a genuine difference in clinical opinion is not necessarily negligent.

Lord Clyde in *Hunter* v. *Hanley*[16] summed this up as follows:

> 'In the realm of diagnosis and treatment there is ample scope for genuine difference of opinion and one man clearly is not negligent merely because his conclusions differ from those of other professional men…The true test for establishing negligence in diagnosis or treatment on the part of a doctor is whether he has been proved to be guilty of such failure as no doctor of ordinary skill would be guilty of if acting with ordinary care.'

In other words, a dentist could not be found negligent if able to demonstrate that where two or more schools of thought existed in a given situation, one of those was followed.

It is possible in the realms of treatment and diagnosis for a dentist to make an error of clinical judgement. A patient may present in pain and a tooth may be extracted. It may in fact be the wrong tooth, but the decision to extract the tooth may not necessarily be negligent. If a body of expert clinical opinion believes that any other

---

Case 1
During enlarging of the mesiobuccal canal of the first molar at the second visit, a file fractured. The patient was immediately informed and a radiograph taken. This showed the fractured instrument to be located very close to the apex of the tooth. The sequelae were discussed with the patient, and the patient given the option of referral to an endodontist to attempt to remove the fractured instrument or, as the instrument was close to the apex, to leave it in situ and complete obturation of the canals. In this case, the dentist's actions were those expected by a responsible body of general dental practitioners; once the event occurred, a radiograph was taken, the likely sequelae discussed with the patient and the option of a referral given.

Case 2
During the enlargement of a canal of a bicuspid, a reamer fractured and a dressing was placed in the chamber. At the following visit, an attempt was made to remove the fractured instrument, using a drill which also fractured. Further enlargement of the access cavity was undertaken to try and remove both pieces. This was unsuccessful. A dressing was placed and a further appointment made. Before the next appointment, the complete crown of the tooth fractured and the patient sought the advice of another dentist, having lost confidence in the first dentist. It was only at this stage, following the taking of a radiograph, that the patient became aware of the fractured instrument. Whilst the initial fracture of the reamer in the bicuspid may not necessarily have been due to negligence, the dentist's subsequent action— failing to inform the patient, not taking a radiograph and not discussing the possible sequelae—may be construed as negligent.

reasonable dentist acting with ordinary care would come to the same conclusions, albeit the wrong ones, given the same radiographs and diagnostic tests, then that dentist will not be found to have acted negligently.

For a dentist, it is comforting to know that you can rely on peers to determine what is an adequate standard of care and that this aspect of a claim is not left to a judge. However, to know that you can rely on a responsible body of dental opinion still involves keeping up to date, knowing the limits of your own expertise and practising within those limits, and seeking further advice or making appropriate referrals whenever you are unsure.

Until recently, the Bolam test meant that as long as the defendant dentist could find a convincing expert to support his actions, the Court was likely to dismiss the allegations made by the claimant. Two things have changed that. The first is the Civil Procedure Rules (1999), which clearly state the role of the expert in clinical negligence cases. Their primary duty is to the court and not to the person who paid them (see Chapter 5). The second is the Bolitho case.[17]

In this tragic case, two-year-old Patrick Bolitho was admitted in January 1984 to St Bartholomew's Hospital in London suffering from croup. He was admitted and later experienced respiratory problems. The case revolved around whether or not he should have been intubated at a certain time on the afternoon of January 16th, earlier than when a cardiac arrest team was summoned. A period of ten minutes elapsed before cardiac and respiratory functions were restored. In that time the lack of oxygen resulted in severe brain damage, and Patrick died shortly after the High Court hearing.

In this case there were two schools of opinion. The claimants' experts gave the opinion that any competent doctor would have intubated Patrick earlier in the afternoon; the defendants' experts thought that intubation was not appropriate. The case went to the House of Lords on appeal from the Court of Appeal, and whilst not finding the doctors negligent in this case, a modification to the Bolam test resulted. Merely having a responsible body of opinion to support the actions of a doctor or dentist is not enough. The professional opinion must be able to withstand logical analysis. Therefore, if a judge finds that the opinion of one expert does not stand up to logic then *Bolitho*

allows him to choose the opinion of the other expert.

> *'The use of these adjectives—responsible, reasonable and respectable—all show that the court has to be satisfied that the exponents of the body of medical opinion relied upon can demonstrate that such an opinion has a logical basis. In particular in cases involving, as they so often do, the weighing of risk against benefits, the judge before accepting a body of opinion as being responsible, reasonable or respectable, will need to be satisfied that, in forming their view, the experts have directed their minds to the question of comparative risk and benefits and have reached a defensible conclusion on the matter.'*

It would be rare that such a situation would arise since experts by their very nature are employed for their skill and knowledge and would not normally be offering views that could not be supported by logic. Nevertheless, the new definition of 'a responsible body of medical opinion' must be that the opinion is logically defensible.

Clinical governance and clinical negligence

Clinical governance as a concept has been with us since 1998, when it was first defined as 'a framework through which NHS organisations are accountable for continuously improving the quality of their services and safeguarding high standards of care by creating an environment in which excellence in clinical care will flourish'.[18] Under the Health Act 1999 [section 18 (1)], for the first time the NHS has a statutory duty 'to put and keep in place arrangements for the purpose of monitoring and improving the quality of healthcare which it provides to individuals'.

Clinical governance has been a 'terms of service' contractual requirement since June 2001 (para 31F National Health Service [General Dental Services, Amendment 9 no.3] Regulations 2001). Every principal/provider dentist is required to have in place a practice-based quality assurance system and to ensure that all members of the practice participate in the programme.

The principles of clinical governance, when applied to general practice, result in:

- clear lines of responsibility for the quality of clinical care
- a comprehensive programme of activity which improves quality
- clear policies for managing risk
- procedures for all healthcare professionals to identify and remedy poor performance.[19]

These systems all help dentists to reduce the chances of errors occurring, improve communication between the patient and the dental team and so in turn reduce successful clinical negligence claims.

The ten pillars of clinical governance are listed in Box 5.1.

Keeping up to date by attending courses, reading professional journals and being involved in peer review and audit are key components of clinical governance. However, the law does not expect a dentist to be aware of every recent development in medical science (*Crawford* v. *Charing Cross Hospital*),[21] but would expect that where a procedure or technique has become 'so well proved' and 'well accepted' then it ought to be adopted.

NICE guidelines

The National Institute for Clinical Excellence was established as a special health authority in February 1999 to give new coherence and prominence to information about clinical guidelines and cost-effectiveness.[22] Clinical guidelines are systematically developed statements which assist in decision making about appropriate healthcare for specific clinical conditions.[23] They are not intended to be a rigid constraint on clinical practice but a distillation of evidence against which the needs of an individual patient can be measured. They sit alongside but do not replace the knowledge and skill of experienced dentists.

Nevertheless, NICE guidelines will assume the credibility of 'a responsible body of opinion' in the eyes of the court, and a practitioner who deviates from them will have to have a very sound and logically defensible reason for deviating from them.

Currently there are only two guidelines published by NICE relating directly to general dental practice — wisdom teeth extractions and recall interval guidelines. (www.nice.org.uk). The importance of complying with the NICE guidelines for impacted wisdom teeth is to avoid unnecessary complications from surgery (such as lingual and ID nerve paraesthesia), to avoid unnecessary general anaesthesia and wasting NHS resources removing caries-free teeth. It also saves wasted time in inappropriate referrals.[24]

The rationale for applying the criteria and risk factors to establish an individual patient's recall interval has more to do with cost effectiveness in the NHS and improving access to NHS services. However, where a patient is not recalled as frequently as necessary to diagnose early changes, the dentist could be vulnerable to a claim if that failure to diagnose leads to damage.

Vocational dental practitioners

Vocational dental practitioners (VDPs) are usually recently qualified dentists who have either worked in house jobs in a dental hospital or come straight from university. Under NHS arrangements, the trainer, who is usually the practice owner, holds a contract with the primary care trust/heath board as a provider. The VDP will work as a performer on the trainer's contract so that any disciplinary action arising out of the VDP's failure to comply with any NHS contractual responsibilities will fall to the trainer.

With regard to a claim in negligence, each VDP is responsible for their own acts or omissions and will not be covered by the trainer. Therefore, it is important that VDPs carry their own professional indemnity.

What is the standard of care expected from VDPs in an NHS training practice? In *Wilsher* v. *Essex Area Health Authority*[25] it was held that the law required a trainee to be judged by the same standard as more experienced colleagues, and that

---

Box 5.1 The ten pillars of clinical governance[20]

1. Evidence based practice
2. Dissemination of good ideas
3. Quality improvement processes in place
4. High quality data to monitor care
5. Clinical risk reduction programmes
6. Adverse risk investigation
7. Lessons learned from patient complaints
8. Poor clinical performance tackled
9. Professional development programmes
10. Leadership skill development.

inexperience could not be a valid defence to clinical negligence. In this particular case involving the administration of excessive oxygen to a premature baby which led to its blindness, the junior doctor was held not to have been negligent because he had taken advice from a senior colleague. In the event, the registrar was found to have been negligent.

This highlights the importance of the supervisory relationship between the VDP and trainer. When a trainer is called in to advise or assist, they assume a duty of care to the patient and it is important they assess the situation for themselves before offering advice or providing treatment, such as locating root canals or embarking on a surgical extraction. Lord Justice Glidwell's judgement in the Wilsher case points to the very real possibility of liability falling on the trainer when reasonable supervision of the vocational training has not occurred, resulting in the negligent act.

The law is clear that the dentist who is inexperienced or who is just learning a particular task or skill must still come up to the standard of a reasonably competent and experienced person. His 'incompetent best' is not good enough (*Nettleships* v. *Weston*).[26] This unforgiving principle takes no account of the particular weaknesses or lack of experience of the dentist but is the law as it currently stands.

> '*In my view, the law requires the trainee or learner to be judged by the same standard of his more experienced colleague. If it did not, inexperience would frequently be urged as a defence to an action for professional negligence*'.

Glidwell LJ in Wilsher *v.* Essex Area Health Authority[27]

Specialists

In the case of specialists, the standard of care is that of a reasonable specialist in that field. The standard is not the best specialist in that field or the most experienced, but that of the 'ordinary' or 'competent' specialist (*DeFreitas* v. *O'Brien*).[28]

CAUSATION

The third and perhaps most important leg of the claim is causation. Once a duty of care has been established and it is proved that the standard of care provided by the dentist fell below that

expected, to prove negligence the claimant has to establish, on the balance of probabilities, that the dentist's negligent act or acts has directly caused the harm or injury for which compensation is being sought.

It is at this hurdle that many claimants' cases fail since it is not enough merely to show that the dentist provided sub-standard care. For example, a poorly completed root canal treatment resulting from a failure to take diagnostic and working length radiographs or any operative measurements may be judged to have been negligently carried out, in that a competent practitioner would be expected to carry out these measurements. However, if the patient has not suffered any damage in terms of pain, loss of function or the requirement to have further treatment, no harm has been *caused* by the negligent act.

The legal burden of proving causation remains upon the claimant and it is not an insubstantial burden, described in some medical contexts as being Herculean (*Chappel* v. *Hart*).[29]

Whilst it may be a stumbling block for claimants, causation is also the unpredictable element from a dentist's point of view and that of the lawyers providing advice, since the application of the concepts of causation and remoteness of damage (whether the damage was the kind that was reasonably foreseeable) is essentially policy driven.

The courts want justice to be done or at least seen to be done, and where damage has occurred and one of the insured parties is in a position to compensate for those damages, then 'where justice and policy demand it a modification of causation principles is not beyond the wit of a modern court' (Lord Steyn in *Chester* v. *Afshar*).[30]

These legal devices are designed to lighten the burdens of the claimant and have been used in the past in a number of cases in the US, Canada and England.

Establishing causation

The difficulty for claimants in clinical negligence cases is to disentangle the causative factors that led to the injury being claimed for. In some cases, the claimant may already be suffering from a disease process long before receiving the alleged negligent treatment, and dental experts called upon to review the issues will sometimes conflict on what is caused by the natural progression of the disease process and what has occurred as a result of the dentist's treatment or failure to treat.

This is a particular aspect of allegations of a failure to diagnose and treat periodontal disease. A patient who has a susceptibility to periodontal disease may allege that the failure to treat the disease has accelerated the loss of those teeth. In establishing causation, the expert would have to decide whether the disease process itself would have led to the loss of those teeth or whether in fact advice and the implementation of a periodontal programme for the patient would have prevented this loss.

Thrown into the melting pot will be the likely host response to these measures at a cellular level, the patient's compliance, habits such as smoking, pre-existing medical conditions and the efficacy of surgical and non-surgical periodontal treatment and published success rates in the round.

Because of the complexity of these factors, the courts are prepared to accept that the claimant has established causation if it can be proved that the negligent act or omission either directly caused or materially contributed to the injury or disease, or materially increased the risk of that injury occurring. Therefore, in the case of periodontal disease, it can be argued that the failure to provide an adequate explanation of the periodontal disease process and give suitable oral hygiene advice has materially contributed to the disease process and increased loss of teeth. It is usually argued by the defendant dentist that the patient was actually provided with this information, but the clinical records sometimes do not reflect this.

Take a case from one of the defence organisations' annual reports.[31] An irregular patient attended for examination, complaining of pain and swelling in the upper right premolar area. A treatment plan was agreed, which involved scaling and filling but no specific investigation of the swollen area was undertaken. Three months into treatment, the patient complained of loose teeth in the quadrant. A radiograph was taken and a diffuse apical lesion noted. A referral was made to a specialist in maxillofacial surgery. A large carcinoma of the palate was diagnosed, necessitating a complete maxillotomy. Whilst the patient obviously had the lesion when she first attended, the late referral had materially contributed to the delay in diagnosis and necessitated the need for a complete maxillotomy as opposed to a hemimaxillotomy, resulting in greater trauma, distress and incapacity for the patient. The case was settled with a sizeable amount of money.

The 'but for' test

In its simplest form, this examination of factual causation tests whether 'but for' the action or inaction of a dentist, damage was caused to the patient or whether in fact the damage was an inevitable result of the consequence of the patient's illness, injury or disease. This is illustrated well by the decision taken in the case below.

Material contribution and material risk

In clinical negligence cases there may be more than one competing cause, any one of which could be responsible for the claimant's condition. However, the claimant does not have to show that the negligence complained of was the only cause of his injury or even the most important one. The threshold of the claimant's success will depend on

---

Barnett v. Chelsea and Kensington Hospital Management Committee[32]

Three night watch men were drinking tea at about 5 a.m. on New Year's Day 1996. Soon afterwards they started vomiting. At about 8 p.m. they presented themselves to casualty. Mr Barnett lay in some chairs whilst another watchman explained their symptoms to a nurse. The nurse telephoned the casualty officer who, himself a little unwell, advised the nurse to tell them to go home and contact their own doctor.

The men left and some hours later Mr Barnett died from what was discovered later to be arsenic poisoning.

The court established firstly that there was a duty of care between the hospital and the deceased claimant, and that the casualty officer had failed in his duty of care in not examining the claimant and admitting him. However, even if Mr Barnett had been admitted, the resulting dehydration and enzyme disturbance already taking place due to the arsenic could not have been reversed, and within the time frame of death occurring the antidote BAL could not have been given.

Therefore, even if the casualty officer had done what he should have done Mr Barnett would still have died, and the case failed on causation.

being able to prove that it made 'a material contribution'.

This was the view taken in *Bonnington Castings* v. *Wardlow*.[33] In a later case, *McGhee* v. *National Coal Board*,[34] the concept of 'material contribution' was equated with 'material risk', so that any action or inaction on the part of a dentist, if it materially increased the risk of the disease or the damage that is being claimed for, would result in a successful claim. Thus, for example, a failure to diagnose caries sufficiently early will materially increase the risk of root canal treatment, which in turn could materially increase the risk of the tooth requiring a cast restoration. Therefore, the claim for damages may include provision of future root canal therapy and a crown, even if the only current remedial treatment is an amalgam restoration.

Loss of a chance

This development in causation was attempted by the courts in *Hotson* v. *East Berkshire AHA*,[35] and whilst it succeeded at trial and at the Court of Appeal, the notion was rejected by the House of Lords. The intention was to say that where a claimant cannot establish, on the balance of probabilities, that the dentist's negligence has led to the damage that is being claimed for, they may be able to establish that due to the dentist's failure they have lost the chance of making a full recovery, or of less damage to occur.

In the Hotson case, a 12-year-old boy fell out of a tree he was climbing during his school lunch hour. He sustained an acute traumatic fracture of the left femoral epiphysis, but on admission to hospital this was not diagnosed. Five days later when he re-presented to the hospital they correctly diagnosed the problem with the hip. The claim was that the failure to diagnose correctly at the first visit had led to avascular necrosis of the epiphysis, which in turn would lead almost certainly to osteoarthritis developing within the joint in the future. The court decided that there was a 75% chance of the vascular necrosis occurring in any case but assessed that the failure to diagnose had denied the claimant a 25% chance that given immediate treatment the necrosis would not have developed.

In dental terms, this can be seen in a failure to diagnose periodontal disease in a patient with pre-existing problems. The claimant could argue that whilst the disease process would have in any case led to the loss of some teeth, the failure to diagnose and treat had led to further avoidable loss, denying the claimant the chance of it not occurring. The House of Lords rejected this 'loss of chance' argument, i.e. that had prompt diagnosis and correct treatment been provided initially, a chance for a better medical result might not have been lost.

Therefore, a claimant must prove their case on the balance of probabilities and would not be entitled to some of the damages if they can only partly prove it in this manner. It remains a matter of policy that a lost chance is not a compensatable damage in clinical negligence cases, and this was affirmed in the Court of Appeal in *Gregg* v. *Scott*.[36]

Chain of causation

A dentist is liable for negligent actions, unless it can be demonstrated that an event unconnected with the original negligence breaks the 'chain of causation'. If that can be established, the defendant either totally escapes liability or the liability is substantially reduced to reflect only that proportion of the claimant's injury that could be attributable to the defendant's negligence.

This new intervening act—*novus actus interveniens*—in terms of causation has to be unconnected with the original negligent event and cannot be foreseeable. For example, in *Sabri–Tabrizi* v. *Lothian Health Board*,[37] the claimant, as a result of a failed sterilisation, became pregnant. The claimant had in fact known that the sterilisation had failed at the time of sexual intercourse and, therefore, the defendant health board was held not to be liable because the chain of causation had been broken.

Defences to medical negligence

Contributory negligence

Whilst it is clear that dentists have a duty of care towards the patients they treat, patients also have certain duties and responsibilities to provide information, follow reasonable instructions and generally to act in their own best interests. The standard to be met would be that of a reasonable patient.

The principles of causation apply to establishing whether the actions or inactions of the claimant have contributed to the injury. Once that has been proved on the balance of probabilities, then either there is a complete defence to the claim, where the claimant is 100% to blame for the injuries in question, or the award for damages will be reduced by an amount decided by the judge.

For example, in the placement of an implant many factors contribute to the success or failure of the osseointegration. Where a claimant has failed to observe post-operative instructions or uses medications, tinctures or other materials around the implant site known to impair healing, or continues to smoke, any failure in the procedure could be attributable to the claimant.

In the one English case in which the claimant's conduct was held to have been negligent (*Pidgeon v. Doncaster*),[38] Pidgeon developed cervical cancer, having been told that the results of her smear test were negative. However, she was held to have been two-thirds contributorily negligent in failing to have a further smear test despite frequent reminders. This is analogous to a patient failing to return for further dental treatment when requested to do so, say after a check-up has revealed pathology on the radiographs.

Failing to seek assistance when it is obvious to any reasonable patient that help should be sought could also amount to contributory negligence, as in the Canadian case of a dental patient who nearly bled to death following an extraction before obtaining medical assistance (*Murrin v. Janes*).[39]

Consent (volenti non fit injuria)

Translated from Latin this means 'no injury is done to a person who consents' (*volens*), and is a general defence in the law of tort. For example, in *Morris v. Murray*[40] the claimant went for a joyride in a light aircraft, knowing that the pilot was very drunk. He was seriously injured when the plane crashed but failed to win any damages as he was held to have consented to run the risk of injury.

The defence of consent is successful if it can be proved that the claimant voluntarily agrees to run the risk of injury. This very much depends on the facts of the case and whether sufficient information was provided to allow the patient to make that decision.

In healthcare, signing a form does not mean the patient is consenting to an act of negligence.

Limitation

This is an important defence to medical negligence and is defined by the Limitation Act 1980. The intention is to limit the time within which a legal claim can be brought against a dentist, as it is well recognised that the longer the time between the alleged act of negligence and the case being brought, the more difficult it is for the parties to mount a case. This is because records may no longer be available or witnesses may be unable to recall the incidents with much clarity.

The Limitation Act defines the primary limitation period as being 3 years from the date on which the cause of action accrued or the date of knowledge if later. The date on which the cause of action accrued is the date of the damage (e.g. when a Dentatus post perforated the root during a core build up). The date of knowledge is when the claimant acquired the knowledge, where 'knowledge' under the Act (section 14 [1]) means knowing:

1. that the injury was significant
2. that the injury was attributable in whole or in part to the act or omission which is alleged to constitute negligence
3. the identity of the defendant.

The identity of the treating dentist can normally easily be gleaned from the records. The real issue is, when did the claimant have actual or constructive knowledge that damage had occurred?

Continuing the example above, the perforated tooth is subsequently used as a bridge abutment. If the dentist does not inform the patient and the tooth remains symptom free for several years, the patient has not yet acquired the knowledge that an injury has occurred. If the patient is then told by another dentist that the perforated tooth is present and this is causing problems, the date of the patient being given that advice is 'the date of knowledge'. The limitation clock starts ticking and the patient has three years from this date within which to issue proceedings. This date of knowledge may in fact be many years after the perforation actually occurred, but the Limitation Act enables the claimant to bring the case.

In *Smith v. Leicestershire Health Authority*,[41] a case of an apparently undiagnosed dermoid cyst pressurising the nerves of the spinal cord, the claimant brought the case some 40 years after the apparent missed diagnosis.

If, on the other hand, the dentist informed the patient at the time of the perforation and went on to give the patient options for its management including referral (and recorded this in the clinical notes), it could be reasonably argued this was the date of knowledge. If this was over three years ago, the Limitation Act could be used as a defence. Equally, the claimant may argue that they did not realise the 'injury was significant' until advised by the new dentist several years later.

Under section 33, the court has discretion to disapply the 3-year rule, taking into account a number of factors including the reasons for the delay and the effect which the delay will have on the quality of the evidence.

In the Smith case above, all the people involved in the event 40 years previously were either dead or so old that they could not reasonably be expected to give evidence. Nevertheless, the Court of Appeal allowed the trial to take place since they argued that the case turned on the radiographs—which were available—and the prejudice to the defendants would be small in relation to that suffered by the claimant if the case was not allowed to proceed to trial.

The case law in relation to limitation is very technical and beyond the scope of this book, but there are a number of texts which deal with this subject (see 'Further reading').

QUANTUM

Quantum is the amount of money that is paid to compensate a claimant for injuries suffered as a result of the dentist's negligence. Compensation figures are not randomly generated but are carefully calculated in relation to the harm caused by the error and what, in financial terms, is required to rectify it. The aim is to try and put the claimant in the position they would have been in had the negligence not occurred.

The court is also able to award punitive damages (called aggravated or exemplary damages) where they believe the clinician has acted maliciously. It is rare in clinical negligence cases but occurred in *Appleton and Others* v. *Garrett*[42] where the dentist was held liable in battery for carrying out unnecessary treatment on healthy teeth.

These figures form the basis of the claimant's case for compensation and form what becomes an integral part of the Letter of Claim and a Part 36 offer.

Compensation payments consist of two parts:

1. **General damages**—for pain, suffering and loss of amenity. The award for loss of amenity covers the claimant's inability to enjoy life in the same way as they could before the accident.
2. **Special damages**—to compensate the patient for specific losses, such as further dental or other treatment required to rectify or alleviate the consequences of negligence, loss of earnings, travel, prescription and medication charges, etc.

The damages payable depend on the facts of the case, and in dental cases most are settled between the parties without proceeding to trial.

The law of damages is meant to be fair to both the claimant and the defendant dentist, and is intended to be limited by what is reasonable. Naturally enough, this element will be keenly contested, but there is one significant UK statutory provision on reasonableness in favour of the claimant. It requires a court to disregard the availability of NHS treatment when determining whether treatment expenses are reasonable. This has the effect of allowing a claimant to seek whatever reasonable remedial treatment they can even if it is in the private sector or provided by a specialist.

Some guidance is available from the Judicial Studies Board (JSB) which records previous settlements (*Guidelines for the assessment of general damages in personal injury cases*),[43] but the defence societies have inevitably built up a wealth of experience in assessing quantum and use this as well as the basis of negotiating settlements.

Claimants also have a duty to mitigate their losses. In *Richardson* v. *London Rubber Company Ltd*,[44] a young couple with two children who did not want any more children were using condoms as their chosen method of contraception. A condom split during use, but the court found that Mrs Richardson had a duty to mitigate her losses (the costs of bringing up an unwanted healthy child) by seeking the morning-after pill. The fact that she did not do so nullified her claim, even if she could prove—which she could not—that the condom had a manufacturer's defect.

CLAIMS FOR CLINICAL NEGLIGENCE

Claims for clinical negligence in dentistry cover a wide range of areas and include the following:

- failure to treat
- failure to diagnose
- diagnostic errors
- failure to take full medical and social histories
- failure to plan treatment appropriately without taking into consideration the patient's occupation
- failure to refer
- failure to utilise special tests including radiographs appropriately
- treatment errors
- warnings not given as appropriate
- post-operative advice and management.

The reader is directed to the annual reports and other risk-management publications produced regularly by the dental defence organisations.

FURTHER READING

Green M, McConnochie K. Clinical negligence and complaints: a clinician's guide. London: Royal Society of Medicine; 2002.

Harpwood V. Negligence in healthcare: clinical claims and risk in context. London: Informa UK; 2001.

McHale J, Fox M, Murphy J. healthcare law: text and materials. London: Sweet & Maxwell; 1997.

Grubb A. Principles of medical law. 2nd edn. Oxford: Oxford University Press; 2004.

Dental Protection Limited. An A–Z of risk management strategies. Annual Review 2000.

REFERENCES

1 Wilson RF, Conrad P, Caparell J et al. Perceived sources of occupational stress in general dental practitioners. Br Dent J 1998; 184: 499–502.

2 Jones M. Medical malpractice in England and Wales: a postcard from the edge. European J of Health Law 1996; 3(2): 109–126.

3 Errors make thousands in hospital even more ill. The Times—16 June 2000.

4 Worried doctors opt for caesareans. The Observer—24 October 2004.

5 Tackling the compensation culture—government response to the Better Regulation Task Force Report—'Better Routes to Redress'. 2004 (www.dca.gov.uk/majrep).

6 Bentley T, Jupp B. Futures for dentistry—the changing environment. London: Demos Organisation; 2000.

7 Donoghue v. Stevenson [1932] AC 562.

8 McLoughlin v. O'Brian [1983] 1 AC 410.

9 Caparo Industries plc v. Dickman [1990] 2 WLR 358.

10 Harpwood V. Negligence in healthcare: clinical claims and risk in context. London: Informa UK; 2001.

11 The Ogopogo [1971] 2 Lloyds Rep 410.

12 Capital Counties plc v. Hampshire CC [1997] 2 All ER 865.

13 Hewlett D, Department of Health. NHS Dentistry: next steps in local commissioning. Department of Health August 2004.

14 Bolam v Friern Hospital Management Committee [1957] 1 WLR 583; [1957] 1 BMLR.

15 Providing protection and peace of mind. Dental Protection Annual Review; 1997.

16 Hunter v. Hanley [1955] SLT 213.

17 Bolitho v. City and Hackney Health Authority [1997] 39 BMLR 1; [1998] Lloyds Rep Med 26.

18 Department of Health. A first class service—quality in the new NHS. Department of Health: London; 1998.

19 Ibid., 32.

20 Rattan R, Chambers R, Wakley G. Clinical governance in general dental practice. Abingdon: Radcliffe Medical Press; 2002.

21 Crawford v. Charing Cross Hospital. The Times—8 December 1953.

22 Department of Health. The new NHS—modern and dependable. London: Department of Health; 1998: para 7.11.

23 Pitts NB. The Scottish inter-collegiate guideline network: guideline 47. Evid-based Dent 2002; 3:93–95.

24 Milner NJ, Smithson NA. Nice Guidelines (letter). Br Dent J 2004; 197(7): 372.

25 Wilsher v. Essex Area Health Authority [1986] 3 All ER 801.

26 Nettleships v. Weston [1971] 2 QB 691, 698, 710.

27 Wilsher v. Essex Area Health Authority [1986] 3 All ER 801.

28 DeFreitas v. O'Brien [1995] 6 Med LR 108.

29 Chappel v. Hart [1998] 72 ALJR 1344 (HC of Aust).

30 Chester v. Afshar [2004] UKHL 41 at 23.

31 Shared Experience. Dental Protection Annual Review; 2003.

32 Barnett v. Chelsea and Kensington Hospital Management Committee [1969] 1 QB 428; [1968] 1 All ER 1068 (QBD).

33 Bonnington Castings v. Wardlow [1956] AC 613.

34 McGhee v National Coal Board [1972] 3 All ER 1008.

35 Hotson v. East Berkshire AHA [1987] AC 750; [1987] 2 All ER 909.

36 Gregg v Scott [2002] EWCA Civ 1471.

37 Sabri–Tabrizi v. Lothian Health Board [1997] 43 BMLR 190.

38 Pidgeon v. Doncaster HA [2002] Lloyds Rep Med 130.

39 Murrin v. Janes [1949] 4 DLR 403 9Nfled TD.

40 Morris v. Murray [1990] 3 All ER 801.

41 Smith v. Leicestershire Health Authority [1996] 36 BMLR 23.

42 Appleton and Others v. Garrett [1997] 8 Med LR 75.

43 Bell R. Judicial Studies Board. Guidelines for the assessment of general damages in personal injury cases. 7th edn. London: Blackstone Press; 2004.

44 Richardson v. London Rubber Company Ltd [2000] Lloyds LR(Med) 280.

Writing reports

6

The role of the expert witness has been thrown sharply into focus by a number of high profile cases. Sally Clark, a solicitor, was freed on appeal in 2003 after the conviction for the murder of her two children was quashed. The expert testimony in this case from Professor Sir Roy Meadow, an expert in sudden infant death syndrome (SIDS), claiming that the chance of a second cot death in a family was 1 in 73 million, was proved to be misleading (the actual figure is closer to 1 in 100 and some research makes it 1 in 4). Dr Williams, a forensic pathologist in this case, also failed to disclose post-mortem blood tests that showed a *Staphylococcus aureus* infection which was probably the more likely cause of death in one of the two children.

In the case against Trupti Patel, who was acquitted of murdering her three babies, Professor Meadow stated that 'one cot death is a tragedy, two is suspicious, three is murder'. Angela Cannings, also freed by the Court of Appeal in 2004, was cleared of killing her two sons. The expert evidence against her was also led by Professor Meadow. A further 258 cases were reviewed by the Criminal Cases Review Commission; 54 of these were still in prison.

Following this case, Lord Justice Judge concluded that: 'If the outcome of the trial depends exclusively, or almost exclusively, on a serious disagreement between distinguished and reputable experts, it will often be unwise, and therefore unsafe, to proceed' unless there was 'additional cogent evidence'. This ruling has already had effects in court.[i]

In 2004, Dr Colin Paterson was struck off by the GMC for giving misleading expert evidence in a number of cases, supporting parents claiming that the apparently abused child had in fact temporary brittle bone disease (TBBD). Associated with this publicity in the press is a growing scepticism about the impartiality of expert witnesses and indeed the very science upon which that expert opinion is based.

A report in *The Times*[1] headlined 'Expert witnesses tempted by cash' quoted Professor Graham Zellick, chairman of the Criminal Cases Review Commission, as saying that high fees tempted experts to give unequivocal opinions just to secure their next case, and some experts appeared to 'make it up as they go along'. Juries, he said, did not always completely understand that experts were only expressing a view. This challenge to the credibility of medical science goes to the very heart of what an expert is expected to do—that is, provide objective opinion to a court of law about the facts and circumstances of a particular case.

Dentists do not often relish the prospect of writing a report with medico-legal implications or appearing in court, but many find themselves doing so in a variety of circumstances. A number of different people or organisations may ask for a report on a patient from a general dental practitioner:

- solicitor
- police
- primary care trust/health board
- disciplinary or regulatory hearing (GDC)
- dentist's employer/practice owner/corporate
- patients.

The first step in writing a report is clarifying your role:

---

[i] In April 2004, Mark Latta was acquitted after being accused of banging the head of his 10-week-old daughter and shaking her, leaving her with 32 fractures and brain damage. Since the experts disagreed as to the cause of death (a common problem in SIDS) the defence argued that since there was no "additional cogent evidence" it was unsafe to convict.

- a lay witness
- a professional witness
- an expert dental witness.

In writing a report it is important that foremost in your mind is the possibility that you may have to explain the report in a court of law. This should concentrate the mind, and certainly if you have any doubts it is worth contacting your defence organisation for advice. Expert witnesses can be held liable for costs if courts believe that an expert has wasted their time because the way in which they gave evidence was unsatisfactory.[2]

Lay witnesses

The role of lay witnesses is simply to tell the court about something they saw or claim to know about a case; they are a witness to a fact. Appearing as a witness to a fact is done in the capacity of a citizen, not as a dentist. An example may be witnessing a fight or the theft of money from the practice by a member of staff. This would be heard in a criminal court—probably a magistrates' court. All criminal cases in England have initial proceedings in the magistrates' court and over 90% are completed there.

A professional witness

A professional witness tells the court factual matters about their patient. In this context, a professional witness may report on the findings following an examination of the patient, the history that was obtained, the clinical diagnosis and findings, and what treatment was provided. This commonly occurs when a patient is treated by a dentist following an injury sustained (e.g. in a road traffic accident, after assault or a fall). In the case of an assault, the dentist is acting as a professional witness of fact but may be asked for an opinion as an expert witness. It is important these distinctions are not blurred, and the dentist should not be tempted to give an opinion outside their field of expertise. For example, being invited to give an opinion as to the *cause* of a particular traumatic dento-alveolar injury may be in the realms of forensic dentistry or a forensic pathologist. Such an offer should be declined unless the dentist can offer an authoritative opinion.

An expert witness

An expert witness is a dentist who will have a claim to a greater level of expertise in a particular field by virtue of training, qualifications and experience. For example, this may be in the field of restorative dentistry, or orthodontics or periodontics. It may also be in general dental practice, for example, where the requirement to establish whether there has been a breach of duty in a particular case needs a like-for-like comparison to care provided by another general dental practitioner.

The specific role of the expert witness is to provide *opinion* on the facts of the case, based on experience and reference to literature. Since it is opinion that is required and the field of dentistry is quite wide, particularly in general practice, it is important for an expert to comment only on matters which lie within the recognised field of expertise.

Second opinion

The increased rise in consumerism is a common theme found in any book on litigation and finds its voice in a request for a second opinion. The nature of dentistry is such that in many circumstances the patient lacks the specialist knowledge needed to make an informed and balanced judgement as to whether the treatment they have received or have been offered is satisfactory. Therefore, patients will present in such circumstances, seeking clarification about a treatment plan or an assessment of treatment that has been carried out.

A patient may request a second opinion in advance of an examination or later in contemplation of legal action against a previous practitioner. In the former case, it is open to the practitioner to decline to provide a second opinion, but the interests of the patient should always be the dentist's first concern. The General Dental Council makes it clear that a patient is entitled to a referral for a second opinion at any time, and the dentist is under an obligation to accede to the request and to do so promptly (GDC Standards for Dental Professionals 1.3).

Patients are entitled to know their dental status, and once a practitioner has examined the patient there is a duty of care to inform them, on a factual basis. This duty of candour does not extend to subjective comments on the quality of the work or diagnosis since without knowing the relevant facts (including problems faced by the previous practitioner at the time) such criticism can only be regarded as inappropriate and possibly misinformed and misleading. These judgemental statements serve neither the interests of patients or the profession at large. Therefore, any written report should be mindful of the potential to be misinterpreted, and only objective, quantifiable and evidence-based statements or inferences must be made.

WRITING THE PROFESSIONAL WITNESS REPORT

A professional witness report may be requested on the dental condition of patients who are already known to a dentist. These requests may come from the police, insurance companies, the Criminal Injuries Compensation Board and other bodies. The format of the reports will vary considerably in their presentation. For example, a witness statement for the police is a section 9 statement under the Criminal Justice Act 1967. The declaration at the top of the statement reads:

'This statement, consisting of x pages, is true to the best of my knowledge and belief and I make it knowing that, if it is tendered in evidence, I shall be liable to prosecution if I have wilfully stated in it anything which I know to be false or do not believe to be true.'

That certainly concentrates the mind.

Requests for reports from solicitors on behalf of their clients should always be accompanied by a signed consent form from the patients allowing the dentist to disclose details from their confidential dental records. In the case of children, consent to reveal information should be given from someone with parental responsibility. Parental responsibility is not always straightforward (see Chapter 2), for example in the case of divorced or unmarried parents. Dental reports have on occasion been requested by couples contesting custody rights over children where oral health

neglect of the child is cited as a reason and the dental report is being used by one or other party to support or deny these allegations.

Organisation of the report

The actual information required by all these reports is essentially the same and the following template headings can be used:

- Your name, address, qualifications, job title, relevant clinical experience and background. A brief CV can be appended to the report if this is a dental expert report.
- Identify the documents, correspondence, instructions and other material (including X-rays) which you have considered as the basis of your report. If records are missing or not available, this should be identified.
- Patient details.
- History.
- Examination — if you have examined the patient confirm the date of the examination, its location and who else was present (e.g. the DSA). In common with such examination reports, subdivide this section into extra oral/intra oral/teeth present, etc. (see Appendix 5 for a specimen layout used by the author in the examination of the patient).
- Radiographic reports.
- Specific comments on expert reports for the other side, or any other documents supplied to you.
- Evaluation of the evidence and/or discussion of the issues.
- Opinion on liability and/or causation (for example).
- Opinion on quantum (where relevant).
- Opinion on prognosis and future treatment needs.
- Date of the report.
- Your signature.
- Expert's declaration (see Appendix 5a).
- Appendix for a glossary of technical terms used—this is important as non-dentists will be reading the report.

The language of the report should be professional and include the appropriate technical terminology. Tooth notation should be explained, but the Palmer tooth notation written as UR6 is easier to understand than the FDI or other system.

Use clear headings so that the facts, opinion and conclusions of the reports can be easily found and read. Often it is the conclusion that a solicitor will read first, and it is important that this conclusion is robust and not influenced by a third party.

A contents page, page numbering and (most important of all) paragraph numbers will make the report easier to navigate. A chronology of events is very useful, and this may take the form of details from the dental records with annotated photographs.

One of the most common problems in expert reports is the blurring of fact with opinion, and dentists should be mindful of this.

SPECIAL KINDS OF REPORT

Condition and prognosis report

For professional and expert witnesses the usual terms of reference for writing reports are 'condition and prognosis'. A claimant has to disclose unilaterally a condition and prognosis report with his Particulars of Claim. Therefore, the purpose is clear-cut, and the expected outcome is a report of the condition of the teeth and what the anticipated future is likely to be. Condition does not just mean the condition of the teeth at the time when they were examined by the expert, but their condition at all times since the commencement of the treatment that is subject of the complaint. Therefore the history is important, and this will include what is provided to you both in written instructions and directly from the patient, as well as previous records.

The present condition of the teeth and oral structures is a factual account, whilst the prognosis of the teeth becomes a matter of opinion based on experience and published evidence. For example, in injuries to front teeth, the likelihood of the loss of vitality is an important consideration depending on the extent of damage, and this should be mentioned in the prognosis section.

The condition and prognosis report should not contain any reference to questions of duty or legal causation. However, it should deal with issues of factual causation and should focus on the aspects of the dentition that are the basis of the claim.

Causation and liability reports

In civil claims, an expert report will comment on causation and liability. The claimant may have one of these reports produced but is under no obligation to disclose it. Breach of duty and causation reports are exchanged simultaneously at a later stage (after the exchange of witness statements of fact).

As discussed in Chapter 5, causation is the direct link between the act or omission and the outcome. Liability is concluded on the basis of the practitioner negligence and whether the standard of care provided has fallen below that expected of another general dental practitioner.

For example, in the case of lingual nerve damage resulting in paraesthesia following the surgical removal of a wisdom tooth, causation may not be in dispute since the two are inextricably linked. It is an entirely different matter as to whether the practitioner has acted negligently and is liable, and factors such as consent, operating technique and warnings will need to be taken into account before making any conclusion on issues about the practitioner's liability.

An important part of the expert's role is providing an opinion but being able to justify any conclusion by reference to the evidence in the case and specialist knowledge. When dealing with an issue on which there is a range of opinion, this must be made clear. Where the expert takes sides in an area of factual dispute, an explanation as to why one version is preferred over the other should be given. The court expects that where there is evidence undermining the expert's opinion, the expert will have discussed it even if a different opinion is favoured. If this other evidence is not mentioned but later raised under cross-examination, the credibility and independence of the expert witness will be compromised.

Quantum

An integral part of assessing the settlement in any civil claim is a quantification of the losses—the quantum. As discussed in Chapter 5, quantum is divided up into general damages and special damages. The special damages are the likely costs of the most appropriate remedial treatment. The costs quoted should reflect the area in which the claimant lives and should find broad acceptance within the profession as a reasonable rate.

APPEARING IN COURT

It is extremely rare for civil claims to end up in court and even less likely in the realms of clinical negligence in dentistry. Therefore, expert witnesses (whilst being prepared for its eventuality) will find most of their activity confined to examining the patient, writing reports, corresponding with solicitors and discussing the case with barristers (counsel) in a case conference. Occasionally, an expert may need to meet face to face with the expert witness from the other side in a formal meeting of the experts.

Where a dentist has produced a professional witness report following, say, an assault, the case may be heard in a magistrates' court where criminal proceeding are taking place. In this case, the dentist may well be asked by the police, via the Crown Prosecution Service, to attend in person as a witness of fact.

As a witness of fact you are called upon to give evidence about what happened in the case, what you recall about the patient, what was said to you and what you did, but not to give opinions. A witness of fact must give oral evidence at the trial unless the opposing parties agree that the witness statement may be read instead. Witnesses of fact may only testify about things that they heard or saw themselves.

The dentist will be able to refer to any contemporaneous records taken and be able to refer to them in the witness box. The statement that was made to the police or solicitors, written some time after the actual event in contemplation of criminal proceedings, is itself not the witness's evidence and, therefore, they are not usually allowed to take the statement into the witness box with them.

Do I have to attend Court?

Dentists are naturally reluctant to attend court. It is both stressful and time consuming for no reward other than a feeling of having done one's duty. Witnesses of fact do not get paid for giving evidence but they can claim travelling expenses.

If required to attend court as part of a trial as a witness, a dentist will be invited to do so by the solicitors. If the dentist fails to reply or refuses to attend court, the solicitors can apply for a witness summons to be issued. This will be served personally, and a witness failing to attend court having received a summons may be arrested, brought to court and fined or imprisoned for failing to comply with a court order.

Where the evidence is uncontested and the witness statement is made under section 9 of the Criminal Justice Act 1967, there is no need for the witness to attend court and the statement can be read out in court. However, where either party objects to the statement being read out because they wish to cross-examine the witness then the dentist must attend in person.

An example of this may be when the dentist claims that the dental injury was caused by a clenched fist or blunt instrument and the defence wishes to challenge this because they believe the victim fell over rather than being assaulted by their client. In this case, the expertise of the dentist to make such statements will be challenged in court under cross-examination. It must be remembered that in a criminal court the burden of proof usually rests on the prosecution to prove every fact in issue beyond reasonable doubt in order to obtain a conviction. This also means disproving the defendant's defence.

The preparation required for appearance in court is beyond the scope of this book, but references to other sources of information are given at the end of the chapter.

EXPERT WITNESS REPORTS

Having discussed general principles in writing reports and detailed the different types, we will now concentrate on the expert witness report. The case law relating to experts is evolving all the time but is based on Part 35 of the Civil Procedure Rules (CPR), and all experts should be familiar with this and the accompanying Practice Direction, as well as the useful Code of Guidance on Expert Evidence (see Appendix 6a and 6b). This is the starting point of understanding the role of the expert in civil cases.

The primary duty of an expert is to report to the court. The expert should be honest and thorough, giving an opinion based on the complete evidence. CPR 35.3 sets out this overriding duty to the court:

1. It is the duty of an expert to help the court on the matters within his expertise.
2. This duty overrides any obligations to the person from whom he has received instructions or by whom he is paid.

In *Gareth Pearce* v. *Ove Arup and Others*,[3] the expert who was an architect produced such a biased report for a fellow architect and so failed in his duty to be independent that the judge felt it necessary to refer his conduct to his professional regulatory body. Mr Justice Jacob said 'at the end of the report the expert said he understood that duty. I do not think he did. He came to argue a case. Any point which might support that case, however flimsy, he took. Nowhere did he stand back and take an objective view as an architect'.

It is this objectivity that is the main requirement of an expert.

Disclosure of reports

Once a report has been produced by an expert there is no compulsion on that instructing party to rely on that report or disclose it to the opposing party. This was confirmed in *Richard Thurber Carlson* v. *Karen Townsend*[4] when a claimant solicitor disclosed a report from an expert whom they had not originally listed to the defendant. Therefore, from an expert's point of view, the decision not to use the report should have no bearing on the cost, and payment to the expert for the report should be made regardless.

In keeping with the expert's duty to the court, all documents sent to the expert for consideration in forming their expert opinion could ultimately be disclosable and, therefore, do not carry legal privilege. An example of this may be copies of counsel's opinion on the pros and cons of the case.

Written questions

Once an expert's report has been disclosed, either party has a right to put written questions to that expert regarding the report, but only for purposes of clarification (CPR 35.6). However, case law would suggest that the scope of questions to experts can be substantial and may involve an attempt to obtain an 'extension' on the views expressed in an expert's report, rather than just 'clarification'.

This was the case in *S J Mutch* v. *Matthew Allen*.[5] In this case, the claimant, Stephen Mutch, was injured in a road traffic accident whilst sitting in the back seat of the car driven by Matthew Allen. Allen alleged contributory negligence because the claimant was not wearing a seat belt. The report produced by the claimant's expert made reference to the fact that a seat belt was not worn but did not indicate the relevance of this to the claimant's injuries. The defendant was allowed to put questions to the expert, and the answers proved damaging to the claimant's case.

On appeal, the questions were deemed to be allowed with the confirmation from the judge that the new regime of CPR 'is designed to ensure that experts no longer serve the exclusive interests of those who retain them, but rather contribute to a just disposal of disputes by making their expertise available to all'.

Meeting of experts and joint statements

Under the provision of CPR Part 35.12, experts are intended to meet to identify the issues in the proceedings and, where possible, reach agreement on an issue. These occur as face-to-face meetings or by telephone, and the usual outcome of a meeting between experts is a 'joint statement' outlining the areas of agreement and disagreement. The experts should not negotiate a conclusion to the matter, nor should they negotiate an answer between two alternative positions to 'split the difference' and arrive at a joint opinion. There is no harm in conceding a point where there is a genuine reason to do so after discussion. The joint statement should detail the areas of agreement and disagreement, with reasons for the difference in opinion. This allows a judge to concentrate on those areas of dispute at the hearing. The joint statement is drawn up between the experts after discussion. One of the experts should agree to draft it since no lawyers should be involved in the process or be in attendance at the meeting of the experts.

Hubbard and Others v. *Lambeth Southwark & Lewisham Health Authority and Others*[6] involved four cases of negligence against a number of doctors crossing six different medical specialities, including paediatric neurology. The importance of a meeting between the experts was clear, and the judge gave further guidance on the advantages and disadvantages of lawyers attending, the biggest disadvantage being the cost, with no real benefit as the lawyers need to be kept out of the debate and the very real risk that if the lawyers for the different sides do become involved they may influence the meeting.

These meetings are privileged and 'without prejudice' in that the parties are not bound by what the experts have discussed and agreed. Nevertheless, the joint statement should be produced very carefully and not disclosed to either party until both experts are happy with it, and it has been agreed and signed by both experts. Once this joint statement is disclosed, it would be very difficult pragmatically for the instructing parties to distance themselves from it, and any agreements or disagreements are likely to be accepted.

Single joint experts

The basis of Lord Woolf's reforms in 1999 of the legal process was to encourage parties to cooperate with each other, save costs, reduce the enormous delays and to introduce the concept of proportionality between the amount of money at stake, the financial position of each party and the complexity of the case. One of the major devices in reducing unnecessary costs and speeding up the process of litigation, when no other forms of resolution are available, was the introduction of the expert who has been appointed and instructed by both parties to the dispute. This fits in well with the essential concept of the expert assisting the court rather than any particular party who instructed or paid them—'an expert should assist the court by providing objective, unbiased opinion on matters within his expertise, and should not assume the role of an advocate' (Practice Direction 1.3).

In clinical negligence cases it is relatively common to use single joint experts in relation to quantum cases where long-term care arrangements are not part of the settlement and peripheral causation points. However, where liability is in dispute, it is still common for each side to instruct their 'own' expert and this was confirmed in *S (a minor)* v. *Birmingham Health Authority*, *Cosgrove* v. *Pattinson* and *Oxley* v. *Penwarden*.[7,8,9]

Cross-examination

The single joint expert's duty is to help the court, and that individual is expected to observe the principles of fairness and transparency so that either party is able to raise issues in relation to the expert report. In *Daniels* v. *Walker*,[10] Lord Woolf indicated that where one of the instructing parties was subsequently unhappy with the report they should first consider whether their concerns could be satisfied by putting questions to the expert submitting the report. The intention is that the report of the single joint expert is the evidence in the case, and that whilst the court may permit cross-examination of the expert to occur either prior to or at the hearing, 'any amplification on cross-examination should be restricted as far as possible'. For the expert there is a certain attraction in being appointed as a single joint expert, since if cross-examination is to be allowed by the court 'then he or she should know in advance what topics are to be covered and where fresh material is to be adduced for his or her consideration…this should be done in advance of the hearing' (*Popek* v. *National Westminster Bank PLC*).[11]

The single joint expert should be instructed jointly by both parties, but where this is not possible 'it is perfectly proper for either separate instructions to be given by one of the parties or for supplementary instructions to be given by one of the parties' (Lord Woolf in *Daniels*)[12]. Both parties should then have equal access to the expert in terms of meetings, and this was confirmed by *Peet* v. *Mid Kent Healthcare NHS trust*.[13]

Liability of the expert witness

One of the concerns for anyone contemplating becoming an expert witness is the issue of liability. This may be in the form of actions for defamation, liability for disciplinary proceeding before the General Dental Council, liability for costs incurred by the instructing solicitors due to poor advice or indeed a late change of mind, and for breach of contract or negligence.

With regard to defamation there is an absolute immunity for all court participants and this is extended to cover all statements made out of court for the purpose of preparing evidence to be given in court. The intention is to allow all those in court to speak freely without fear that 'any disgruntled or possibly impecunious persons against whom they gave evidence might subsequently involve them in costly litigation' (*Marrinan* v. *Vibart*).[14] This core immunity for an expert witness 'in essence relates to the giving of evidence' (*Darker and Others* v. *Chief Constable of West Midlands Police*)[15] but does not extend to the fabrication of evidence, in this case a written report of a police interview of the suspect containing fabricated admissions.

In the case of *Stanton* v. *Callaghan*,[16] the claimant's expert made a significant concession at the experts' meeting, resulting in the acceptance by the claimant's party of a modest settlement. In order to recover their cost, the solicitors who instructed the expert then started proceedings against the expert. This case concluded that the expert has immunity for being sued if the claim is based on evidence in court, a report deployed at the hearing and possibly the exchanged report. This was because it was felt that an expert's duty should be received 'in an atmosphere free from threats of suit from disappointed clients'. This case thus confirmed that in civil cases, an expert has immunity from a lawsuit from a party who has instructed the expert and whose report they were relying on for exchange with the other side, even if the expert did not subsequently give evidence in court. This immunity will cover the expert report, and any subsequent reports or clarifications of the evidence contained in the reports.

This is significant because it allows an expert (when discussing the case at a meeting of the experts) to make concessions where appropriate without fearing that any departure from previous opinion will be seen as negligent. As Chadwick LJ says in *Stanton*, 'The immunity is needed in order to avoid the tension between a desire to assist the court and fear of the consequences of a departure from previous advice'.

This was further clarified in *Rais* v. *Paimana*[17] by the judge: 'One reason underlying immunity is that there should be no undue inhibition upon a witness being prepared to revise his earlier statement if he subsequently recognises it to be wrong, for whatever reason, or to need qualification'.

However, there will be no such immunity for the expert if the claim made against them is based on a report advising on merits of the client's case when given early in the litigation process. This was further confirmed in *Palmer* v. *Durnford Ford*:[18] an expert who carries out work for the main purpose of giving advice to the client, rather than for the purpose of disclosure to the other side, does not have immunity.

For a general dental practitioner this is quite relevant, as the judgement in *Hughes* v. *Lloyds Bank PLC*[19] confirms. The claimant wished to sue the estate of her general practitioner, as the GP had prepared a report indicating that following a road accident the claimant's condition was not serious. As a result of the report, the claimant accepted a relatively meagre offer for general damages. The claimant's condition was actually more serious than the GP had indicated, and she sued him for his negligent prognosis. The Court of Appeal allowed the action to continue on the basis that the GP's report had been prepared to assist in preliminary negotiations with the insurers, and there was no indication that the report would have been used had the litigation proceeded.[20] This case is important for dentists who produce reports for their own patients who have been injured, since they could be held liable if their prognosis for any particular teeth is less than accurate. It is advisable that dentists check with their indemnity organisations that this aspect of their work is covered.[ii]

Whilst in court, the expert is immune from any claim. 'A witness owes no duty of care to anyone in respect of the evidence he gives in court. His only duty is to tell the truth' (*Hall* v. *Simons*).[21]

The future of witness immunity may be in doubt following the decision on advocates' immunity in *Hall* v. *Simons*, and there may be further assaults on witness immunity in the future since there has been a trend towards curtailing or

---

[ii] A press release from Dental Protection dated 14/12/04 confirmed that members were covered for expert reports as they are an integral part of the practice of dentistry. The same cover is applied by Dental Protection to dentists who are involved in committee work, advisory/consultancy work or representative roles.

abolishing 'as of rights' immunity in this area of the law. Current interpretation of the law of precedent in this area, as it stands, confirms that expert's immunity from a lawsuit remains intact.

Payment for expert reports

It is difficult to give recommended charges for the production of expert reports, since, just as in general practice, individual overheads differ. However, what is important is to draw up 'terms and conditions of engagement', within which will be:

- the hourly rate charged for examining the patient, writing the report, meeting counsel and other experts
- fees for attendance in court
- charges for travelling
- fees for cancellation of a court attendance up to 10 working days before the date of the hearing.

The Expert Witness Institute and the Academy of Experts both have model terms and conditions on their websites.

The Civil Procedure Rules enable the court to limit the amount of experts' fees and expenses that the party wishing to rely on the expert may recover from any other party (CPR 35.4(4)). Therefore, experts would be well advised to ensure that their terms of business provide for any court-imposed limitations on their fees to be met by those instructing them.

FURTHER READING

Available:
http://www.medicalprotection.org/assets/pdf/booklets/reports_gps_essential.pdf.
The Academy of Experts. CPR Code of Guidance for Experts and those instructing them. Online. Available: http://www.academy-experts.org/cpr v2.0 July 2004.
Bond C, Solon M, Harper P, Burn S. The expert witness in court: a practical guide. 2nd edn. Crayford: Shaw; 1999.
Expert Witness Institute. The Law and You: code of guidance on expert evidence. Expert Witness Institute. Online. Available: http://www.ewi.org.uk/practice.asp.
Medical Protection Society. Writing reports and giving evidence in court: an essential guide for GPs. MPS Medico-legal Advice 003. London: Medical Protection Society; 2002. Online.
A Practical Guide to the use of Expert Witnesses. Smith and Williamson 2002.

REFERENCES

1 The Times. 30 November 2004.
2 Expert witnesses 'now liable for court costs'. Hospital Doctor 2 Dec 2004.
3 Gareth Pearce v Ove Arup Partnership Limited [2001] EWHC Ch 455.
4 Richard Thurber Carlson v. Karen Townsend [2001] EWCA Civ 511.
5 S J Mutch v. Matthew Allen [2001] EWCA Civ 76.
6 Hubbard and Others v. Lambeth Southwark & Lewisham Health Authority and Others [2001] EWCA Civ 1455.
7 S (a minor) v. Birmingham Health Authority. The Times: November 23 1999.
8 Cosgrove v. Pattinson [2001] All ER (D).
9 Oxley v. Penwarden [2001] Ll Med Rep 347 (CA).
10 Daniels v. Walker [2000] 1WLR 1382.
11 Popek v. National Westminster Bank PLC [2002] EWCA Civ 42.
12 Daniels v. Walker [2000] 1WLR 1382.
13 Peet v. Mid Kent Healthcare NHS trust [2001] EWCA Civ 1703.
14 Marrinan v. Vibart [1963] 1 QB 234.
15 Darker and Others v. Chief Constable of West Midlands Police [2001] 1 AC 435.
16 Stanton v. Callaghan [1999] 2 WLR 745.
17 Rais v. Paimana [2000] QB PAA 252.
18 Palmer v. Durnford Ford [1992] 2 QB 483.
19 Hughes v. Lloyds Bank plc [1998] PIQR P98.
20 A Practical Guide to the use of Expert Witnesses. Smith and Williamson 2002.
21 Hall v. Simons [2000] 3 WLR 543.

Appendices

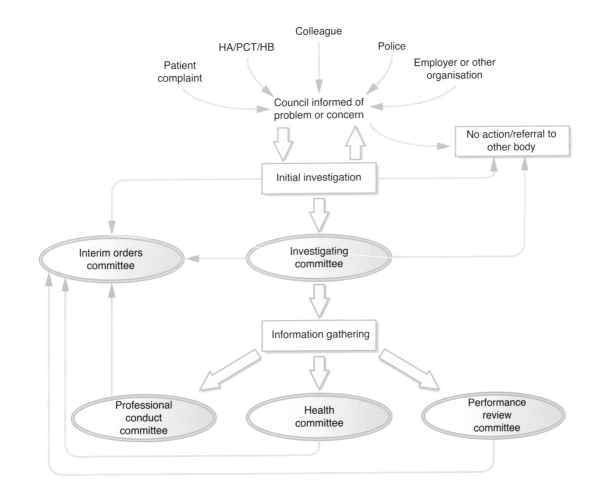

APPENDIX 2   RECORD AUDIT – COMPLETENESS

Patient	1	2	3	4	5	6	7	8	9	10
Patient contact details										
Medical history										
Tobacco/alcohol use										
Medical alerts										
Dental history										
Existing restorations										
Carious lesions										
Perio status/BPE										
Other soft tissue status										
Occlusal info										
Radiographic report										
Diagnosis										
Treatment plan										
Consent/options recorded										
Signed and dated notes										

APPENDIX 3   AUDITS OF RADIOGRAPHIC IMAGE QUALITY

The Guidance Notes for Dental Practitioners on the Safe Use of Equipment (Department of Health, NRPB 2001) recommend a simple, subjective quality rating system to be used for dental radiographs as follows:

Rating	Quality	Basis
1	Excellent	No errors of patient preparation, exposure, positioning, processing or film handling
2	Diagnostically acceptable	Some errors of patient preparation, exposure, positioning, processing or film handling, but which do not detract from the diagnostic utility of the radiograph
3	Unacceptable	Errors of patient preparation, exposure, positioning, processing or film handling, which render the radiograph diagnostically unacceptable

Based on the above quality rating, audit targets to improve performance can be set. Suitable targets the legislation suggests should be met, in relation to the overall percentage of radiographs taken by the practice and individual dentists, are as follows:

Rating	Target
1	Not less than 70%
2	Not less than 20%
3	Not greater than 10%

APPENDIX 4   QUICK REFERENCE: ACCESS TO HEALTH RECORDS CHECKLIST[i]

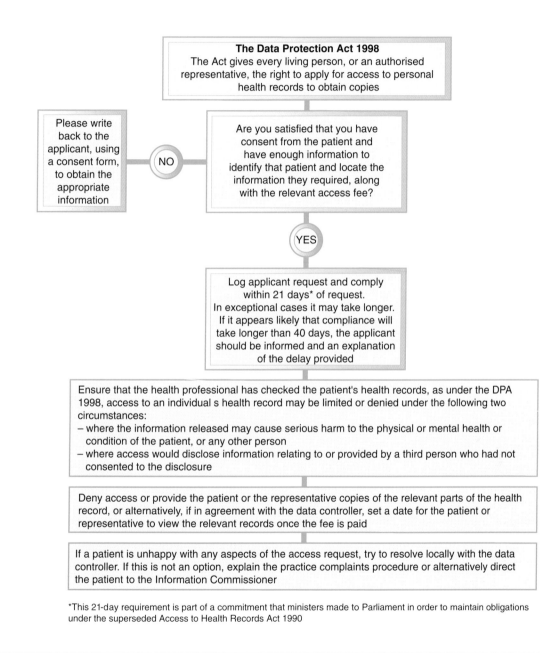

The Data Protection Act 1998
The Act gives every living person, or an authorised representative, the right to apply for access to personal health records to obtain copies

Please write back to the applicant, using a consent form, to obtain the appropriate information

NO

Are you satisfied that you have consent from the patient and have enough information to identify that patient and locate the information they required, along with the relevant access fee?

YES

Log applicant request and comply within 21 days* of request.
In exceptional cases it may take longer.
If it appears likely that compliance will take longer than 40 days, the applicant should be informed and an explanation of the delay provided

Ensure that the health professional has checked the patient's health records, as under the DPA 1998, access to an individual s health record may be limited or denied under the following two circumstances:
– where the information released may cause serious harm to the physical or mental health or condition of the patient, or any other person
– where access would disclose information relating to or provided by a third person who had not consented to the disclosure

Deny access or provide the patient or the representative copies of the relevant parts of the health record, or alternatively, if in agreement with the data controller, set a date for the patient or representative to view the relevant records once the fee is paid

If a patient is unhappy with any aspects of the access request, try to resolve locally with the data controller. If this is not an option, explain the practice complaints procedure or alternatively direct the patient to the Information Commissioner

*This 21-day requirement is part of a commitment that ministers made to Parliament in order to maintain obligations under the superseded Access to Health Records Act 1990

[i] From: 'Guidance for Access to Health Records request under the Data Protection Act 1998. Department of Health; 2001.

APPENDIX 5 GENERAL DENTAL COUNCIL GUIDANCE ON PRINCIPLES OF CONFIDENTIALITY[ii]

Our core standards guidance *Standards for Dental Professionals* sets out six key principles which you should apply to all aspects of your work as a dental professional.

It is your responsibility to apply the principles to your daily work, exercising your judgement in the light of the principles.

The guidance states:

'Protect the confidentiality of patients' information'.

- Treat information about patients as confidential and only use it for the purpose for which it is given.
- Prevent accidental disclosure or unauthorised access to confidential information by keeping information secure at all times.
- In exceptional circumstances, disclosure of confidential patient information without consent may be justified in the public or patient's interest. Seek appropriate advice before disclosing information on this basis.

You have both an ethical and a legal duty to keep patient information confidential. This guidance deals with the ethical issues around protecting the confidentiality of patients' information.

We do not give legal advice. As *Standards for Dental Professionals* explains, you are responsible for making yourself aware of laws and regulations which affect your work, premises, equipment and business, and complying with them. If you are in doubt on the legal issues around protecting and providing patient information, ask an appropriate source—for example, your defence organisation—for advice.

Duty of confidentiality

- Patients are entitled to expect that you will protect the confidentiality of information you hold about them.
- Confidentiality is central to the relationship of trust between you and your patient.

- The duty of confidentiality applies:
  - to all members of the dental team
  - to all information about the patient which you learn in your professional capacity and from which the patient can be identified. This includes, for example, recognisable patient images such as photographs.
- The duty of confidentiality applies even after a patient dies.
- If it is necessary to disclose patient information:
  - Seek the patient's consent to do so wherever possible. Read our guidance *Principles of Patient Consent* for advice on obtaining consent.
  - Make sure that you only disclose the minimum information necessary for the purpose.
  - Be prepared to justify your decisions and any action you take.

Disclosure with the patient's consent

- Make sure that you explain to patients the circumstances in which information about them might be shared with others involved in their healthcare.
- Give patients the opportunity to withhold permission for you to share information about them.
- Where a patient allows you to share information about them, make sure the patient understands:
  - what you will be disclosing
  - the reasons you will be disclosing it
  - the likely consequences of the disclosure.
- If you have permission to disclose information, make sure anyone you share that information with understands that the information is confidential.
- If you are given patient information to enable you to provide care for a patient you have a legal duty to keep the information confidential.
- You may be asked to provide patient information by third parties, for example, to assist teaching or research, or you may yourself wish to use patient information for the purposes of teaching or research. If so, make sure you apply the principles in this guidance by:

[ii] This was published in June 2005

- seeking the patient's consent, whether or not you judge that the patient can be identified from the disclosure
- making sure the patient understands exactly what they are consenting to and how the information will be used
- making sure that you only disclose the minimum information necessary for the purpose.
- If it is not necessary for the patient to be identified from the disclosure, anonymise the data you disclose so that the patient cannot be identified.

Preventing accidental disclosure

- Make sure that you protect the confidential information you are responsible for when you receive it, store it, transmit it or dispose of it.
- Store records securely and don't leave them lying around or on screen where they might be seen by other patients, unauthorised health care staff or members of the public.
- Don't talk about patients where you can be overheard.

Disclosure in the 'public interest'

- You may judge that you should share confidential information without consent in the public interest. This might happen where the patient puts their health and safety or other people's health and safety at serious risk.
- If you think it is in the public interest for you to share confidential information, before you act, and where practicable, do everything you can to persuade the patient to disclose the information themselves, or to give you permission to disclose the information.
- If you cannot persuade the patient to do this, or it is not practicable to do so, take advice from an appropriate source, such as your defence organisation, before you disclose the information.

Disclosure required by court order

- A court may order you to disclose patient information without consent. If so:
  - Take legal advice from an appropriate source such as a defence organisation before you disclose the information.
  - Only disclose the minimum information necessary to the proceedings.
- In any circumstance where you decide to disclose confidential information, be prepared to explain and justify your decision and any action you take.

APPENDIX 6 GENERAL DENTAL COUNCIL GUIDANCE ON OBTAINING CONSENT

Our core standards guidance *Standards for Dental Professionals* sets out six key principles which you should apply to all aspects of your work as a dental professional.

It is your responsibility to apply the principles to your daily work, exercising your judgement in the light of the principles.

The guidance states:

'Respect patients' dignity and choices'.

- Treat patients with respect and courtesy, in recognition of their dignity and rights as individuals.
- Recognise and promote patients' responsibility for making decisions about their bodies, their priorities and their care, making sure you do not take any steps without consent.

It is a general legal and ethical principle that valid consent must be obtained before starting treatment or physical investigation, or providing personal care, for a patient. This principle reflects the right of patients to determine what happens to their own bodies, and is a fundamental part of good practice.

Patients have a right to choose whether or not to accept your advice or treatment. This guidance expands on the ethical principles of obtaining patient consent which you should apply to your work.

We do not give legal advice. As *Standards for Dental Professionals* explains, you are responsible for making yourself aware of laws and regulations which affect your work, premises, equipment and business, and complying with them. If you are in doubt on the legal issues around obtaining patient consent, ask an appropriate source—for example, your defence organisation—for advice.

Ethical issues in obtaining patient consent

- You should give patients the information they want and need, in a way they can use, so that they are able to make informed decisions about their care.
- Giving and obtaining consent is a process, not a one-off event. It should be part of an ongoing dialogue between you and the patient.
- For consent to be valid, the patient must have received sufficient information to make the decision.

- Take steps to find out what your patients want to know as well as telling them what you think they need to know. Examples of information which patients should know or may want to know include:
  - why you think a proposed treatment is necessary
  - risks and benefits of proposed treatment
  - what might happen if the treatment is not carried out
  - any alternative forms of treatment available, and their risks and benefits
  - details of anticipated treatment costs.

Explaining costs

- In respect of costs, you should always make clear to the patient:
  - the nature of the contract and in particular whether the patient is being accepted for treatment under the NHS or privately
  - the charge for an initial consultation and the probable cost of subsequent treatment.
- Where treatment is likely to be extensive, give the patient a written treatment plan and estimate.
- If, having agreed an estimate with the patient, you think that you will need to modify the treatment plan, make sure you obtain the patient's consent to any further treatment and additional cost; and give the patient an amended written treatment plan and estimate.

Informed consent

- Giving a patient clear information to enable them to take a decision may involve using written material, visual or other aids to best explain aspects of treatment.
- Try to meet particular communications needs such as hearing difficulties or language barriers, for example, by suggesting that the patient brings a friend who can sign or interpret if there are hearing or language difficulties, or providing a hearing 'loop'.
- Satisfy yourself that the patient has understood the information you have given them.
- Consider whether they would like more information before making a decision; and whether they would like more time before making a decision.
- Respond honestly and fully to any questions the patient has.

- Involve other members of the dental team in discussion with the patient, where appropriate. They may have valuable knowledge about the patient's background and particular concerns.
- Do not pressurise the patient to accept your advice. The decision must be that of the patient.
- Patients have a right to refuse consent to investigation or treatment. If they do so, they also have a right to expect that doing so will not negatively affect their relationship with you.
- Once given, a patient may withdraw consent at any time, including during the performance of a procedure.
- Make sure that, once consent has been obtained, the patient is given a clear route for reviewing the decision with the person providing the treatment.
- Make sure you are clear as to the scope of the authority the patient has given you. For example, whether the patient consents to all or only part of a proposed treatment plan.

Who obtains consent?

- If you are the member of the dental team providing the treatment it is your responsibility to discuss it with the patient and obtain consent as you will have a comprehensive understanding of the procedure or treatment, how it is carried out and any risks attached to it. If it is not practicable for you to obtain consent, you may delegate these tasks provided you ensure that the person to whom you delegate:
  - is suitably trained and qualified
  - has sufficient knowledge of the proposed treatment
  - understands the risks involved
  - follows the principles explained in this booklet.
- If you delegate the responsibility of obtaining consent, you will remain responsible for making sure, before you start any treatment, that the patient has been given sufficient time and information to make an informed decision, and has given consent to the procedure or investigation.

Capacity to give consent

- Every adult has the right to make his/her own decisions and must be assumed to have capacity to do so, unless demonstrated otherwise. Where there is any doubt, assess the capacity of the patient to give informed consent by considering whether or not the patient understands and can weigh up the information necessary to make the decision in question.
- Consult your defence organisation or a professional body for up-to-date advice on:
  - how to deal with an adult patient who you think lacks capacity to give informed consent
  - the law in relation to the capacity of children to give informed consent.

APPENDIX 7   EXAMINATION OF PATIENT – FOR USE IN WRITING REPORTS

Note that if during your examination of the patient there is something wrong with that patient that needs further attention, such as undiagnosed pathology, the expert has a duty of care to inform the patient and advise the patient's general dental practitioner. This is best done by a separate letter. Below is an examination pro forma for writing reports.

DENTAL REPORT

Claimant's name: _____

Date of accident: _____

Date of examination: _____

Circumstances of accident: _____

_____

_____

Dental injuries sustained: _____

_____

_____

TREATMENT

Immediate: _____

_____

Subsequent and ongoing: _____

_____

Past dental history of relevance: _____

_____

_____

SOCIAL: Smoking _____

Alcohol _____

Contact sports _____

MEDICAL HISTORY: _____

_____

_____

EXAMINATION

Extra-oral

Lips _____

TMJ _____ Left _____ Clicking/Pain _____
                                 Right _____ Clicking/Pain _____

Muscles _____

Opening _____ Width _____
                                Deviation _____

Aesthetics: high/low lipline _____

Intra-oral

Lips _____

Soft tissue _____

Tongue _____

FOM _____

Palate _____

Teeth present

      Charting on records card _____

Occlusion

      Incisal relationship _____

      Wear _____

      Anterior guidance _____

      Working side/Non-working side interference _____

      Canine guidance _____ Left _____
                                      Right _____

Perio

      Pocket charts/recession/OH

Traumatic injuries

      Tests _____

      Vitality tests _____

      Transillumination _____

      Percussion _____

      Mobility _____

Future treatment needs _____

Prognosis _____

APPENDIX 8 DECLARATION BY EXPERT AT END OF REPORT

I understand that my duty in writing this report is to help the Court on matters within my expertise; I understand this duty overrides any obligation to the person(s) from whom I have received instructions or by whom I am paid.

I confirm that I have complied with that duty in writing my report.

I believe the facts I have stated in the report are true and the opinions I have expressed are correct.

APPENDIX 9 CIVIL PROCEDURE RULES: PART 35 EXPERTS AND ASSESSORS

This can be found on the Department of Constitutional Affairs website at www.dca.gov.uk/civil/procrules_fin/contents/parts/part35.htm

Contents of this part

Duty to restrict expert evidence

35.1 Expert evidence shall be restricted to that which is reasonably required to resolve the proceedings.

Interpretation

35.2 A reference to an 'expert' in this Part is a reference to an expert who has been instructed to give or prepare evidence for the purpose of court proceedings.

Experts – overriding duty to the court

35.3 (1) It is the duty of an expert to help the court on the matters within his expertise.

(2) This duty overrides any obligation to the person from whom he has received instructions or by whom he is paid.

Court's power to restrict expert evidence

35.4 (1) No party may call an expert or put in evidence an expert's report without the court's permission.

(2) When a party applies for permission under this rule he must identify –

(a) the field in which he wishes to rely on expert evidence; and

(b) where practicable the expert in that field on whose evidence he wishes to rely.

(3) If permission is granted under this rule it shall be in relation only to the expert named or the field identified under paragraph (2).

(4) The court may limit the amount of the expert's fees and expenses that the party who wishes to rely on the expert may recover from any other party.

General requirement for expert evidence to be given in a written report

35.5 (1) Expert evidence is to be given in a written report unless the court directs otherwise.

(2) If a claim is on the fast track, the court will not direct an expert to attend a hearing unless it is necessary to do so in the interests of justice.

Written questions to experts

35.6 (1) A party may put to –

(a) an expert instructed by another party; or

(b) a single joint expert appointed under rule 35.7,

written questions about his report.

(2) Written questions under paragraph (1) –

(a) may be put once only;

(b) must be put within 28 days of service of the expert's report; and

(c) must be for the purpose only of clarification of the report,

unless in any case –

    (i) the court gives permission; or

    (ii) the other party agrees.

(3) An expert's answers to questions put in accordance with paragraph (1) shall be treated as part of the expert's report.

(4) Where –

(a) a party has put a written question to an expert instructed by another party in accordance with this rule; and

(b) the expert does not answer that question,

the court may make one or both of the following orders in relation to the party who instructed the expert –

    (i) that the party may not rely on the evidence of that expert; or

    (ii) that the party may not recover the fees and expenses of that expert from any other party.

Court's power to direct that evidence is to be given by a single joint expert

35.7 (1) Where two or more parties wish to submit expert evidence on a particular issue, the court may direct that the evidence on that issue is to be given by one expert only.

(2) The parties wishing to submit the expert evidence are called 'the instructing parties'.

(3) Where the instructing parties cannot agree who should be the expert, the court may –

(a) select the expert from a list prepared or identified by the instructing parties; or

(b) direct that the expert be selected in such other manner as the court may direct.

Instructions to a single joint expert

35.8 (1) Where the court gives a direction under rule 35.7 for a single joint expert to be used, each instructing party may give instructions to the expert.

(2) When an instructing party gives instructions to the expert he must, at the same time, send a copy of the instructions to the other instructing parties.

(3) The court may give directions about –

(a) the payment of the expert's fees and expenses; and

(b) any inspection, examination or experiments which the expert wishes to carry out.

(4) The court may, before an expert is instructed –

(a) limit the amount that can be paid by way of fees and expenses to the expert; and

(b) direct that the instructing parties pay that amount into court.

(5) Unless the court otherwise directs, the instructing parties are jointly and severally liable (GL) for the payment of the expert's fees and expenses.

Power of court to direct a party to provide information

35.9 Where a party has access to information which is not reasonably available to the other party, the court may direct the party who has access to the information to –

(a) prepare and file a document recording the information; and

(b) serve a copy of that document on the other party.

Contents of report

35.10 (1) An expert's report must comply with the requirements set out in the relevant practice direction.

(2) At the end of an expert's report there must be a statement that –

(a) the expert understands his duty to the court; and

(b) he has complied with that duty.

(3) The expert's report must state the substance of all material instructions, whether written or oral, on the basis of which the report was written.

(4) The instructions referred to in paragraph (3) shall not be privileged (GL) against disclosure but the court will not, in relation to those instructions –

(a) order disclosure of any specific document; or

(b) permit any questioning in court, other than by the party who instructed the expert, unless it is satisfied that there are reasonable grounds to consider the statement of instructions given under paragraph (3) to be inaccurate or incomplete.

Use by one party of expert's report disclosed by another

35.11 Where a party has disclosed an expert's report, any party may use that expert's report as evidence at the trial.

Discussions between experts

35.12 (1) The court may, at any stage, direct a discussion between experts for the purpose of requiring the experts to –

(a) identify and discuss the expert issues in the proceedings; and

(b) where possible, reach an agreed opinion on those issues.

(2) The court may specify the issues which the experts must discuss.

(3) The court may direct that following a discussion between the experts they must prepare a statement for the court showing –

(a) those issues on which they agree; and

(b) those issues on which they disagree and a summary of their reasons for disagreeing.

(4) The content of the discussion between the experts shall not be referred to at the trial unless the parties agree.

(5) Where experts reach agreement on an issue during their discussions, the agreement shall not bind the parties unless the parties expressly agree to be bound by the agreement.

Consequence of failure to disclose expert's report

35.13 A party who fails to disclose an expert's report may not use the report at the trial or call the expert to give evidence orally unless the court gives permission.

Expert's right to ask court for directions

35.14 (1) An expert may file a written request for directions to assist him in carrying out his function as an expert.

(2) An expert must, unless the court orders otherwise, provide a copy of any pro-posed request for directions under paragraph (1) –

(a) to the party instructing him, at least 7 days before he files the request; and

(b) to all other parties, at least 4 days before he files it.

(3) The court, when it gives directions, may also direct that a party be served with a copy of the directions.

Assessors

35.15 (1) This rule applies where the court appoints one or more persons (an 'assessor') under section 70 of the Supreme Court Act 1981[1] or section 63 of the County Courts Act 1984.[2]

(2) The assessor shall assist the court in dealing with a matter in which the assessor has skill and experience.

(3) An assessor shall take such part in the proceedings as the court may direct and in particular the court may –

(a) direct the assessor to prepare a report for the court on any matter at issue in the proceedings; and

(b) direct the assessor to attend the whole or any part of the trial to advise the court on any such matter.

(4) If the assessor prepares a report for the court before the trial has begun –

(a) the court will send a copy to each of the parties; and

(b) the parties may use it at trial.

(5) The remuneration to be paid to the assessor for his services shall be determined by the court and shall form part of the costs of the proceedings.

(6) The court may order any party to deposit in the court office a specified sum in respect of the assessor's fees and, where it does so, the assessor will not be asked to act until the sum has been deposited.

(7) Paragraphs (5) and (6) do not apply where the remuneration of the assessor is to be paid out of money provided by Parliament.

---

[1] 1981 c.54.

[2] 1984 c.28. Section 63 was amended by S.I. 1998/2940.

APPENDIX 10 CIVIL PROCEDURE RULES: PRACTICE DIRECTIONS—EXPERTS AND ASSESSORS

This practice direction supplements CPR part 35.

This can be found on the Department of Constitutional Affairs website at

www.dca.gov.uk/civil/procrules_fin/contents/ practice_directions/pd_part35.htm.

Contents of this Practice Direction

Expert evidence—general requirements
Form and content of expert's reports
Information
Instructions
Questions to experts
Single expert
Assessors

Part 35 is intended to limit the use of oral expert evidence to that which is reasonably required. In addition, where possible, matters requiring expert evidence should be dealt with by a single expert. Permission of the court is always required either to call an expert or to put an expert's report in evidence.

Expert evidence – general requirements

1.1 It is the duty of an expert to help the court on matters within his own expertise: rule 35.3(1). This duty is paramount and overrides any obligation to the person from whom the expert has received instructions or by whom he is paid: rule 35.3(2).

1.2 Expert evidence should be the independent product of the expert uninfluenced by the pressures of litigation.

1.3 An expert should assist the court by providing objective, unbiased opinion on matters within his expertise, and should not assume the role of an advocate.

1.4 An expert should consider all material facts, including those which might detract from his opinion.

1.5 An expert should make it clear:

(a) when a question or issue falls outside his expertise; and

(b) when he is not able to reach a definite opinion, for example because he has insufficient information.

1.6 If, after producing a report, an expert changes his view on any material matter, such change of view should be communicated to all the parties without delay, and when appropriate to the court.

Form and content of expert's reports

2.1 An expert's report should be addressed to the court and not to the party from whom the expert has received his instructions.

2.2 An expert's report must:

(1) give details of the expert's qualifications;

(2) give details of any literature or other material which the expert has relied on in making the report;

(3) contain a statement setting out the substance of all facts and instructions given to the expert which are material to the opinions expressed in the report or upon which those opinions are based;

(4) make clear which of the facts stated in the report are within the expert's own knowledge;

(5) say who carried out any examination, measurement, test or experiment which the expert has used for the report, give the qualifications of that person, and say whether or not the test or experiment has been carried out under the expert's supervision;

(6) where there is a range of opinion on the matters dealt with in the report –
  (a) summarise the range of opinion, and
  (b) give reasons for his own opinion;

(7) contain a summary of the conclusions reached;

(8) if the expert is not able to give his opinion without qualification, state the qualification; and

(9) contain a statement that the expert understands his duty to the court, and has complied and will continue to comply with that duty.

2.3 An expert's report must be verified by a statement of truth as well as containing the statements required in paragraph 2.2(8) and (9) above.

2.4 The form of the statement of truth is as follows:

'I confirm that insofar as the facts stated in my report are within my own knowledge I have made clear which they are and I believe them to be true, and that the opinions I have expressed represent my true and complete professional opinion.'

2.5 Attention is drawn to rule 32.14 which sets out the consequences of verifying a document containing a false statement without an honest belief in its truth.

(For information about statements of truth see Part 22 and the practice direction which supplements it.)

Information

3 Under Rule 35.9 the court may direct a party with access to information which is not reasonably available to another party to serve on that other party a document which records the information. The document served must include sufficient details of all the facts, tests, experiments and assumptions which underlie any part of the information to enable the party on whom it is served to make, or to obtain, a proper interpretation of the information and an assessment of its significance.

Instructions

4 The instructions referred to in paragraph 2.2(3) will not be protected by privilege (see rule 35.10(4)).

But cross-examination of the expert on the contents of his instructions will not be allowed unless the court permits it (or unless the party who gave the instructions consents to it). Before it gives permission the court must be satisfied that there are reasonable grounds to consider that the statement in the report of the substance of the instructions is inaccurate or incomplete. If the court is so satisfied, it will allow the cross-examination where it appears to be in the interests of justice to do so.

Questions to experts

5.1 Questions asked for the purpose of clarifying the expert's report (see rule 35.6) should be put, in writing, to the expert not later than 28 days after receipt of the expert's report (see paragraphs 1.2 to 1.5 above as to verification).

5.2 Where a party sends a written question or questions direct to an expert, a copy of the questions should, at the same time, be sent to the other party or parties.

5.3 The party or parties instructing the expert must pay any fees charged by that expert for answering questions put under rule 35.6. This does not affect any decision of the court as to the party who is ultimately to bear the expert's costs.

Single expert

6 Where the court has directed that the evidence on a particular issue is to be given by one expert only (rule 35.7) but there are a number of disciplines relevant to that issue, a leading expert in the dominant discipline should be identified as the single expert. He should prepare the general part of the report and be responsible for annexing or incorporating the contents of any reports from experts in other disciplines.

Assessors

7.1 An assessor may be appointed to assist the court under rule 35.15. Not less than 21 days before making any such appointment, the court will notify each party in writing of the name of the proposed assessor, of the matter in respect of which the assistance of the assessor will be sought and of the qualifications of the assessor to give that assistance.

7.2 Where any person has been proposed for appointment as an assessor, objection to him, either personally or in respect of his qualification, may be taken by any party.

7.3 Any such objection must be made in writing and filed with the court within 7 days of receipt of the notification referred to in paragraph 6.1 and will be taken into account by the court in deciding whether or not to make the appointment (section 63(5) of the County Courts Act 1984).

7.4 Copies of any report prepared by the assessor will be sent to each of the parties but the assessor will not give oral evidence or be open to cross-examination or questioning.

APPENDIX 11 IRISH LAW

Introduction

This section examines certain specific differences between Irish law and the general legal principles discussed in the body of the text. In general, such differences are few; the broad brushstrokes of the law in the UK and the Republic of Ireland (referred to as 'Ireland' in the text that follows) are similar, reflecting the common origins of their legal systems. However, in some areas, especially when it comes to institutional structures and legal systems, the differences are sufficiently great to require that they be flagged and discussed.

Here we discuss the main distinctions under the following headings:

- Legal systems
- Regulation
- Consent
- Negligence
- Expert witnesses.

Legal system

There is an important backdrop to Irish law which is lacking from its UK counterpart, namely the existence of a written Constitution. The Constitution is the foundational legal document of the Irish State and delineates institutional structures, roles of the various arms of government and the rights of individuals. No law can be passed that is in violation of the Constitution, and no institution can exercise powers that are not given to it by the Constitution. For example, the Irish Constitution contains an explicit description of how general elections are to take place. No law could be passed to change that system unless the Constitution itself were first amended. Similarly, the Constitution is the basis for a principle that only judges can sit in judgement of legal cases with far-reaching consequences: this has practical consequences for the regulation of the profession, to which we return below.

Save for the Constitution (and it is a very large difference), the Irish legal system, with its hierarchy of courts, its distinction between public and private law, its reliance on both statute and common law for legal guidance, and the burgeoning influence of European legislation is broadly similar to that in the UK.

Regulation and governance

There are—as matters presently stand—no bodies in Ireland equivalent to the NHS or NICE, although reforms are in place that will create a Health Service Executive (replacing the Health Board system) with national responsibility for delivery of publicly-funded healthcare. Compared with the UK, a far higher proportion of dentists are self-employed and are therefore not answerable to any form of employing authority.

The regulatory body for Irish dentists is the Dental Council, which was brought into being by the Dentists Act 1985. As in the United Kingdom, its regulatory role is predominantly twofold. Firstly, it is responsible for the execution and maintenance of a Register of Dental Practitioners and no person may practise as a dentist who is not on that register. Secondly, it has responsibility for investigating complaints made to it; such complaints can come from the public, from other professionals, or may be generated by the Council itself. The Fitness to Practise (FTP) Committee of the Council is the ultimate arbiter of misconduct. When a complaint is made to the Council, it is the FTP Committee that decides whether the complaint is of sufficient gravity. If it is not, the Council will be advised of that fact, although the Dental Council can disagree with the FTP Committee's finding and direct that an enquiry be held. Where the FTP Committee feels that a complaint is of sufficient gravity then an enquiry is held.

Any FTP enquiry will be concerned with whether either or both of two criteria are satisfied:

1. whether the dentist is guilty of professional misconduct
2. whether the dentist is unfit to practise by reason of some physical or mental disability.

The FTP enquiry takes the form of a hearing in which the case against the dentist is presented (typically by a lawyer on behalf of the Council) and in which the dentist (also legally represented) presents his case. Witnesses are examined and cross-examined under oath, just as in a court and the Council has the power to compel the attendance of witnesses and to order the production of documents. If the FTP finds against a dentist then its findings are presented to the Council and it may pursue one of a number of courses:

- warning as to future conduct
- censure of the practitioner
- attachment of conditions to continuing practice
- suspension of the practitioner from the register for a period of time
- striking the practitioner off the register.

We noted above that the Irish Constitution stipulates that it is the role of judges to make serious decisions on questions of fact, where those decisions will have far-reaching consequences for a person's future. Accordingly, where the Dental Council recommends that a practitioner be suspended from or struck off the register, then the decision must be ratified by the Irish High Court. Only then does it have the force of law. The dentist will have the opportunity to make representations to the High Court before any order is ratified or (where there has been some alleged error by the Council) to apply to the High Court for judicial review of the disciplinary decision.

Consent

The law on consent in Ireland is again broadly similar to that in the United Kingdom. Consent must meet these three indispensable criteria:

1. Consent should be voluntary.
2. Consent should be given by someone with the capacity to do so, in terms of both age and cognitive function.
3. Consent should be based on sufficient relevant information.

The text has already dealt with the broad issues of consent (see Chapter 3). However, in respect of 1 and 2 above, Irish law has shades of difference from its UK counterpart: we look here at the issue of consent by minors and the question of so-called 'informed consent'.

Consent and minors

The law for 16- and 17-year-olds is clear in Ireland. Section 23 of the Non-Fatal Offences against the Person Act 1997 makes clear that a person over the age of 16 years can give valid consent to medical, dental and surgical treatment. It is worth noting that the same section does not explicitly give 16- and 17-year-olds the capacity to refuse treatment, but it is broadly accepted that they would have the power to do so in most cases.

The question of treating minors under the age of 16 is not so clear-cut. While the law on 'competent minors' is well established in the UK, 'Gillick competence' has never been formally endorsed in Ireland. Again, this is in part a function of the Irish Constitution, which specifically accords great deference to the nuclear family as the building block of Irish society. Irish law affords parents a greater role in a child's life than might be the case in other countries, the net effect of which is that it cannot be said with certainty that minors under the age of 16 can be treated without their parents' consent. It does appear clear that parents can decide on behalf of their children only insofar as their decisions will not pose a serious threat to the life or health of a child. Hence, parents have been permitted to refuse routine diagnostic tests on behalf of their infant children (*North Western Health Board* v. *W(H)* [2001] 3 IR 635) but have not been permitted to refuse blood transfusions necessary to preserve life.

In general, the state of Irish law is that it would always be preferable to obtain parental consent prior to treating children under the age of 16 years. The Irish Dental Council's guide to *Professional Behaviour and Dental Ethics* bears out that the consent of a parent or guardian should be sought for those under the age of 16. However, the same document also states (at paragraph 3.10): 'It should be noted that persons under the age of 16 years can validly withdraw consent given by a parent/guardian.' It is not clear to the author that this is an accurate statement of the law: if children under 16 are not generally competent to *give* consent, they are probably not competent to *refuse* it without parental agreement. The same capacity is, in broad terms, required for both consenting to treatment and refusing treatment. It does not seem to make sense that where parents give consent for their 11-year old child to undergo necessary dental treatment, that child would be free to negate that parental consent. If that were the case, why would one not seek consent from the child in the first place? However, it seems clear that this provision is not intended to apply to such young minors and rather reflects the need to take account of the wishes of the older minor in circumstances where his wishes conflict with those of his parents. Although this does not express the law in Ireland, it highlights the direction the law should perhaps take and is, in any event, eminently practical advice.

Informed consent

When consent is given by a patient, that patient's consent is only valid if the patient has been given sufficient information to make his decision. The question then arises: what is 'sufficient' information? The two competing perspectives are sometimes termed the 'doctor-centred' test and the 'patient-centred' test.

In the 'practitioner-centred' test, the patient has sufficient information when given as much information as the reasonable practitioner would give in the circumstances. In other words, a dentist who fails to tell a patient everything relating to a treatment would not be negligent, so long as a reasonable quantity of information had been disclosed (see Chapter 5). The 'reasonableness' of this disclosure will be measured by reference to what another practitioner of equal skill and status would have disclosed. The Irish Supreme Court has endorsed this 'practitioner-centred' approach to informing consent (*Bolton* v. *Blackrock Clinic*, unreported Supreme Court). There are some qualifications to this test and we return to them below.

In the 'patient-centred' test, sufficient information is disclosed once the dentist has told the patient what the reasonable patient would wish to know in the circumstances. So, according to this test, a dentist could not rely on withholding information merely because the 'reasonable practitioner' would have done so in circumstances where that information is something the 'reasonable patient' would have wished to know (whether or not the reasonable practitioner would have disclosed it). The reason why the 'reasonable patient' approach is relevant in Ireland is because one recent High Court decision (concerning dental treatment) has suggested that the reasonable patient test is the approach that should be taken by Irish law in future (*Geoghegan* v. *Harris* [2000] 3IR 536). It is possible that, when next asked to consider the matter, the Irish Supreme Court might well agree with this approach.

A practical approach to informed consent

Because the Supreme Court outranks the High Court, Irish law is still best expressed by the decision in the *Bolton* case. What this means is that a dentist will not be negligent in obtaining consent if he has disclosed such information that is in accordance with a reasonable comparable dental practice. However, it is important to augment this statement with reference to the fact that the Supreme Court in the *Bolton* case appeared to add two riders to the Irish law of informed consent:

1. Where an intervention is elective, there is probably a higher onus of disclosure on the dentist. In other words, in emergency dental surgery, fewer risks may be disclosed, whilst in a cosmetic procedure a fuller picture of potential risks must be painted.
2. Whenever a procedure carries a risk of pain extending into the future and requiring treatment or further procedures, then that risk (however remote) should be disclosed.

Furthermore, it will always be prudent for the practitioner to take into account any information that would not usually be disclosed but about which the patient wishes to know. This requirement is expressed in the Dental Council guide to *Professional Behaviour and Dental Ethics*:

> Good communications with patients are essential and dentists should be prepared to answer patients' questions openly and honestly and in terms the patient can understand.

The greater the disclosure in any event, the less room there is for doubt about whether the patient was properly informed.

Negligence

The test for clinical negligence in Ireland is broadly similar to that in the UK and was most clearly summarised in the case of *Dunne* v. *National Maternity Hospital*. The test(s) can be paraphrased as follows:

1. A dentist is negligent when guilty of such failure as no practitioner of equal status and skill would be guilty of if acting with ordinary care.
2. If the allegation of negligence is that the dentist deviated from a general and accepted practice, then that alone will not amount to negligence unless the course the practitioner took was one that no reasonable practitioner would have taken.

3. Conversely, even if the dentist can show that the approach taken is one that is endorsed by professional practice, that dentist may still be negligent if the course taken is one that has inherent defects obvious to anyone giving the matter due consideration.

4. A simple difference of opinion between practitioners as to which is the better of two ways of treating a patient cannot provide the basis for saying that one or other must have been negligent.

5. The matter will not be decided by the judge's opinion as to which of two approaches is preferable, but by the judge's assessment of medical evidence as to what a careful comparable practitioner would or should have done.

The practical consequences of this are that in order not to be negligent, a dentist must follow courses of action that are consistent with 'reasonable' practice. The approach need not be universal (indeed, how could it be, if dental practice is to develop new techniques and approaches) or even the majority view, but it must be a reasonable thing to have done or to have omitted to do in all the circumstances. A negligence case is decided on the basis of independent expert evidence: if Dr A is accused of negligence, it is likely that she will rely on the evidence of a comparable dental practitioner to the effect that her conduct was in accordance with a body of responsible dental opinion. The plaintiff in the case will be required to call expert dental evidence to say that Dr A's conduct

was inconsistent with any reasonable body of dental practice. It will be a matter for the judge in the case to decide which is the more persuasive testimony.

Expert evidence

There is—regrettably, to many people's minds—no equivalent of the Woolf reforms in Irish law. Where a case turns on expert clinical evidence, it is open to all parties (and there may be very many of them where there are multiple plaintiffs and/or defendants) to seek expert reports and to submit those reports as evidence. Accordingly, a dentist may be retained 'for' either the defendant or the plaintiff. However, being retained in this way does not diminish the dentist's over-riding duty of impartiality: the expert is there to help the court and not to help the plaintiff or defendant to win the case.

Any report that is sought to bolster or quantify a legal claim and which is to be used in legal action for personal injuries in the High Court must be exchanged with the other side. So, any report that is prepared by a dentist for such a case will be seen by the other side prior to the day of the trial. In cases in the lower courts, reports are also typically exchanged.

Recommended reading

Mills S. Clinical practice and the law. Dublin: Butterworths; 2002.
Madden D. Medicine, ethics and the law. Dublin: Butterworths; 2002.

APPENDIX 12 SCOTTISH ISSUES ON CONSENT

The general approach of Scots law to the issue of consent for medical and dental care is very similar to its treatment in England and Wales. Indeed, one would not expect a significant variation in approach across jurisdictions. Decisions taken by the Courts of England and Wales, though persuasive rather than binding in Scotland, have been influential in the development of the law of consent in Scotland. However, there are notable areas where there is a divergence in approach, and with which practitioners will require to be conversant.

Assault

Chapter 3 reviewed the potential for the offence of battery being committed in England and Wales where treatment is undertaken without consent. The Scottish equivalent to battery is 'assault'. In terms of the common law of Scotland, assault is both a crime that can be subject to a criminal prosecution, and a civil wrong that can found a remedy in damages.

There are no reported decisions of prosecutions being taken against medical/dental practitioners for performing treatment without consent, and this may be seen as a recognition that well-intentioned medical intervention will not be punished as a criminal offence. The position would be different where unnecessary treatment is deliberately performed.

In Scotland, it is almost unheard of for damages to be sought for assault. Establishing consent will, of course, provide a defence to such a claim. The only reported case comes from the late nineteenth century when a prisoner sought to recover damages from a doctor on the basis that the doctor had committed an assault by inoculating a patient against his will. The claim was not upheld, and it appears that the court construed that the patient had consented to the procedure. The standard approach remains for patients to bring an action for damages against their treating practitioners on the basis of professional negligence, but nevertheless Scots law does afford patients the opportunity to bring their claim for damages on the basis that they have been subject to an assault. This approach may find favour with patients who have been subject to malevolent or unnecessary treatment.

Capacity of children to consent to dental treatment in Scotland

Scotland has its own legislation addressing the capacity of children and young people to consent to medical treatment. The governing statute is the Age of Legal Capacity (Scotland) Act 1991. Broadly, the Act provides that legal capacity is acquired at age 16. However, there are exceptions to that general rule. The relevant provision relating to consent to medical and dental treatment is found in Section 2(4) which provides as follows:-

'A person under the age of 16 years shall have legal capacity to consent on his own behalf to any surgical, medical or dental procedure or treatment where, in the opinion of a qualified medical practitioner attending him, he is capable of understanding the nature and possible consequences of the procedure or treatment.'

It is notable that the test to be applied in assessing capacity for those under 16 is a subjective one to be taken by the treating doctor or dentist. The test is a specific statutory one, which does not invoke the concept of what would be in the best interests of the child. A child under 16 years will have legal capacity if the dentist conducting a procedure or treatment holds the opinion that the child is capable of understanding the nature and possible consequences of that procedure or treatment.

Consequently, young persons attending a dentist who are aged 16 or over will have capacity to consent to or refuse dental treatment. Effectively, Scots law views such individuals as adults.

If a person is under 16, the dentist must apply the abovementioned test and reach an opinion on whether the patient is capable of understanding the nature and possible consequences of the procedure or treatment proposed. It is of note that under separate legislation, the Children (Scotland) Act 1995 Section 6, there is a presumption that a child aged 12 or more will be of sufficient age and maturity to form a view on decisions concerning them, though it has to be emphasised that being able to form a view does not necessarily mean that one has capacity to provide consent. So, a dentist will be able to treat a child aged under 16 with their consent if the dentist is satisfied that the child understands the nature and consequences of the treatment proposed. If the dentist considers that the child does not have that necessary understanding, consent to the procedure will require to be obtained from a parent or guardian of the child.

It is notable that the test provides for a child under 16 to have legal capacity to consent to treatment, but that the provision does not expressly extend to a child having capacity to refuse consent to treatment. Unfortunately, there remains uncertainty on this point, though it appears that the consensus view amongst commentators is that the capacity to consent would extend also to capacity to refuse treatment. This in turn raises the question as to whether a parent or guardian can consent to treatment for a child which the child has refused. The practical solution may be for the dentist to conclude that in these circumstances the child does not have the necessary understanding of the recommended treatment or procedure for them to have capacity to make decisions on their treatment.

It should be stressed that this issue has not been canvassed before the Courts in Scotland and as such there is no definitive guidance on the capacity of children under the age of 16 to refuse to consent to medical treatment or procedures. In England, the courts have intervened to override the refusal to consent of young persons under the age of 16 (*re M (child): refusal of medical treatment)* [1999] 2 FLR1097); a decision taken exclusively on the basis of child's best interests.

Parental responsibility

When children under 16 years do not have the necessary capacity to consent to medical treatment, consent can be given by someone who has parental responsibilities and rights for the child. Where both parents of a child have parental rights then only the consent of one is required. This mirrors the position in England and Wales.

Parental rights in Scotland broadly follow the position in England. As such:

- All mothers acquire parental responsibilities and rights on the birth of a child.
- If the parents are married at the time of conception or subsequently then both parents have parental responsibilities and rights.
- If the parents are unmarried then only the mother has parental responsibilities and rights.

The unmarried father will have parental responsibilities and rights by agreement with the child's mother or by court order.

- A very wide class of persons are entitled to apply to the court for an order relating to parental rights under the Children (Scotland) Act 1995; these have included unmarried fathers, grandparents, sperm donors and step-parents.
- A child's guardian will have parental responsibilities and rights.
- Local authorities may take responsibility for a child by virtue of a parental responsibilities order; this removes parental responsibilities and rights from the child's parents.

Section 5 of the Children (Scotland) Act 1995 extends the category of person who can consent to medical or dental treatment for a child. A person aged 16 or over who has 'care or control of a child' under 16 can consent to treatment where the child is not able to give their own consent, and it is not within the knowledge of the person that a parent of the child would refuse to give the consent in question.

Section 6 requires the person giving consent to have regard so far as practicable to the views of the child and anyone who has parental responsibilities or rights for them.

Adults with incapacity

In cases of temporary incapacity, for example where a patient is unconscious, then a medical practitioner is entitled to act according to necessity and in the patient's best interests. This broadly follows the position in England and Wales.

However, in situations of permanent incapacity the Scottish position is governed by the Adults with Incapacity (Scotland) Act 2000, one of the first pieces of legislation to be enacted by the Scottish Parliament. The Act provides a framework for dealing with the property, financial affairs and personal welfare of incapable adults. Part 5 of the Act deals with the medical treatment of adults who are incapable of giving consent. For the purposes of Part 5, 'medical treatment' includes 'any procedure or treatment designed to safeguard or promote physical or mental health' and therefore includes dental treatment.

The Act requires that if a dentist or other medical practitioner is of the view that a patient lacks the capacity to consent to treatment, then authority to treat must be obtained. In most cases the authority must be obtained from the medical practitioner with primary responsibility for the patient's general medical care. Usually this will be the patient's GP.

The authority is contained in a certificate in which the medical practitioner must state that he is of the opinion that the adult is incapable in relation to a decision about the medical treatment in question. The certificate shall specify that such authority will only exist for a period which the medical practitioner considers appropriate to the patient's condition, and not exceeding one year from the date of the examination which prompted the certificate to be granted.

In some situations, patients may have a welfare guardian appointed; in this event consent should be obtained from the guardian. Where there is disagreement between the medical practitioner and guardian with regard to the treatment of the adult, the medical practitioner is required to consult with the Mental Welfare Commission in order to have a 'nominated medical practitioner'

appointed in order to adjudicate and provide opinion on the proposed treatment.

Where the adjudicating medical practitioner has consulted the guardian and is of the opinion that the treatment should be given, the patient's medical practitioner may then administer it. If the adjudicating medical practitioner is of the opinion that the treatment should not be given, the patient's medical practitioner may apply to the Court of Session in order to determine whether the proposed treatment should be administered.

The Scottish Executive's Code of Practice for persons authorised to carry out medical treatment or research under Part 5 of the Act makes specific reference to situations where a delay in treatment may put the adult at risk. There, the existing common law authority for a doctor to treat a patient in order to prevent loss of life or a serious deterioration in condition is referred to, with that authority not being superseded by any provision of the 2000 Act.

The figure below sets out the basic scheme of the Adults with Incapacity (Scotland) Act 2000 with regard to dental care.

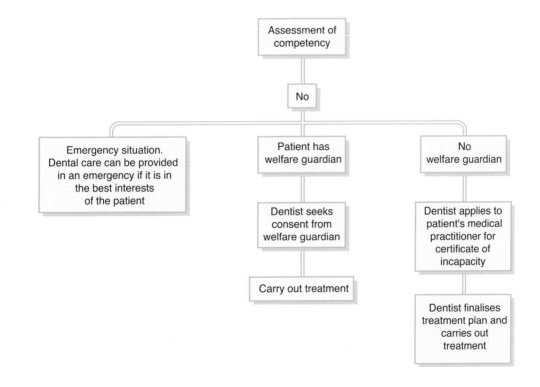

Index

Page numbers in bold refer to boxes, figures or tables. This index also contains full details of case law and legislation.